HEART RATE TRAINING

ROY BENSON
DECLAN CONNOLLY

Human Kinetics

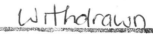

Library of Congress Cataloging-in-Publication Data

Benson, Roy.
  Heart rate training / Roy Benson, Declan Connolly.
    p. cm.
  Includes index.
  ISBN-13: 978-0-7360-8655-4 (soft cover)
  ISBN-10: 0-7360-8655-2 (soft cover)
  1. Cardiovascular fitness. 2. Heart rate monitoring. I. Connolly,
Declan, 1965- II. Title.
  QP113.B46 2011
  616.1'05--dc22

                              2010046982

ISBN-10: 0-7360-8655-2 (print)
ISBN-13: 978-0-7360-8655-4 (print)

Acquisitions Editor: Laurel Plotzke Garcia; **Developmental Editor:** Cynthia McEntire; **Assistant Editor:** Elizabeth Evans; **Permission Manager:** Martha Gullo; **Copyeditor:** Patsy Fortney; **Indexer:** Dan Connolly; **Graphic Designer:** Bob Reuther; **Graphic Artist:** Tara Welsch; **Cover Designer:** Keith Blomberg; **Photo Asset Manager:** Laura Fitch; **Art Manager:** Kelly Hendren; **Associate Art Manager:** Alan L. Wilborn; **Illustrations:** © Human Kinetics; **Printer:** McNaughton & Gunn

Human Kinetics books are available at special discounts for bulk purchase. Special editions or book excerpts can also be created to specification. For details, contact the Special Sales Manager at Human Kinetics.

Printed in the United States of America   10 9 8 7 6 5 4 3 2 1

The paper in this book is certified under a sustainable forestry program.

Human Kinetics
Web site: www.HumanKinetics.com

United States: Human Kinetics
P.O. Box 5076
Champaign, IL 61825-5076
800-747-4457
e-mail: humank@hkusa.com

Canada: Human Kinetics
475 Devonshire Road Unit 100
Windsor, ON N8Y 2L5
800-465-7301 (in Canada only)
e-mail: info@hkcanada.com

Europe: Human Kinetics
107 Bradford Road
Stanningley
Leeds LS28 6AT, United Kingdom
+44 (0) 113 255 5665
e-mail: hk@hkeurope.com

Australia: Human Kinetics
57A Price Avenue
Lower Mitcham, South Australia 5062
08 8372 0999
e-mail: info@hkaustralia.com

New Zealand: Human Kinetics
P.O. Box 80
Torrens Park, South Australia 5062
0800 222 062
e-mail: info@hknewzealand.com

E4932

Cheers, Dr. Z.

Dr. Z is a diligent scientist, an engaging scholar, a fitness enthusiast, a critical thinker, and a compassionate and understanding man. He epitomizes a mentor. Thank you, Dr. Z. We hope our work here reflects both your work and humor.

CONTENTS

Acknowledgments **vii** • Introduction **ix**

PART I   **Foundations**   **1**

CHAPTER 1   Monitoring for Maximum Performance . . . **3**

CHAPTER 2   Evaluating and Customizing Your Zones . . **21**

CHAPTER 3   Getting the Most From Your Monitor. . . . **37**

PART II   **Training**   **43**

CHAPTER 4   Targeting Sport-Specific Fitness
With Heart Rate **45**

CHAPTER 5   Increasing Aerobic Endurance **53**

CHAPTER 6   Raising Anaerobic Threshold **67**

CHAPTER 7   Boosting Speed and Power **85**

INTRODUCTION

Congratulations! You're about to learn why heart rate monitoring is one of the most convenient and most effective ways to train. You're on your way to becoming better conditioned in a more time-efficient manner. When you understand your heart rate, learn how to measure it, and have a reliable monitor, you are on your way to a scientifically designed exercise program, individualized just for you, that will guarantee results.

The main problem with most exercise programs is that they are not based on your unique body shape, size, physiological response, and most important, current fitness level. They aren't designed just for you. In fact, it's likely these exercise programs have little to do with you. For the most part, they are generic programs based on basic exercise physiology. They come in the form of classes, training groups, clubs, or books written by self-styled experts. But despite the quality of the teaching and the validity of the general principles, they don't answer the "What about me?" question. Often, you can't figure out how to apply the information to yourself. Everyone who wants to exercise, get in shape, or train has the same dilemma: "Should I run? Take a spinning class? Use the rowing machine? Just swim?" Once the choice is made, the next question is, "Yes, but what about *me*? How do I go about this? Now that I've picked something, how far, how fast, how hard, how often should *I* go?"

The *what* question is not hard to address. We hope that you've picked something that is convenient, looks like fun, or seems the easiest. The *how* question usually is the stumper.

Do what you want and call it what you will, but your effort has to be *individualized*. It must be based on your current fitness level, general ability, and goals. The simplest way to create an individualized program is to track your cardiac response to your body's movement of choice. Then you can observe the adaptations that reflect your responses and no one else's.

The good news is that modern technology has produced a wide selection of affordable heart rate monitors. They provide instant, reliable feedback about your body's response to your chosen exercise and intensity. Whether you are a beginner, intermediate, or advanced athlete, there is a heart rate monitor for you with all the bells and whistles you need.

Heart Rate Training will guide you through the necessary steps to help you realize three goals:

1. Find the best way to make a heart rate monitor work for you.
2. Learn to apply the principles of exercise physiology to get in the best possible shape.

3. Combine these two goals to benefit from training that is totally individualized to your ability, fitness level, and goals.

To help you meet the first goal, we share our collective wisdom from years of working with heart rate monitors and doing research. We offer tools and ideas we've developed. We show you how to be sure your numbers are reliable and how to interpret what they tell you about yourself.

To help you meet the first and second goals, we dispel some of the confusion and answer the most common questions that come up regarding heart rate training. The first challenge to address is the confusion in the popular literature about heart rate training zones. One article may claim that to get in shape, you should train at a certain percentage of your maximum heart rate. The next article notes that you should work out in a certain percentage zone of your maximum oxygen uptake capacity, often expressed as percentage of $\dot{V}O_2max$ or written out as a percentage of your maximum volume of oxygen uptake. Because both of these suggestions are valid, we combine them to make it as easy as possible to calculate your target heart rate. This solution appears in chapter 1.

A further challenge in meeting the second goal has to do with the lingo used in both the lab and the locker room. Unfortunately, no laws regulate the words used to communicate about exercise, physical fitness, or workouts. It is simply a matter of semantics, and unfortunately, neither academia nor the general population has reached unanimous agreement about the vocabulary. Rather than present lab vocabulary or dictionary definitions, we prefer to use the language most commonly found in the popular literature. First, we focus on just two aspects related to the response of your heart to the need for oxygen: aerobic and anaerobic conditioning. In addition, although many other terms are used by authorities, writers, and athletes to refer to and define other physical capacities developed while working toward peak shape, we talk primarily about four components of physical fitness: endurance, stamina, economy, and speed.

Accomplishing goal 3 is a cinch when you use a heart rate monitor because it allows you to perfectly individualize your training. The principles are broad, but your response is as narrow as your ability, shape, and goals require.

This book is organized progressively. First, it presents the relevant background and basic exercise science you need to know to understand training. Chapters 1 through 7 cover some basic physiological adaptations, equipment issues, and other information regarding your training and fitness. The next chapters progress into the various adaptation stages you'll go through. Finally, we present a selection of exercise programs for walking, jogging, running, cycling, triathlon, swimming, rowing, and cross-country skiing. The final chapter covers using heart rate in the training of team sport athletes. These programs contain different levels, or intensities, to cater to individual fitness abilities and goals.

PART I

FOUNDATIONS

CHAPTER 1

Monitoring for Maximum Performance

This chapter introduces the concept of heart rate monitoring and explains how to monitor it accurately to get the specific adaptations you want. The first step, then, is to identify those adaptations. They are the four main components of fitness: endurance, stamina, economy, and speed. Because these components are interdependent, they must be developed in a progressive manner. The heart rate approach will allow you to stay in the target zone for the correct amount of time and prevent you from the all-too-common problem of overreaching, or overtraining. Once you understand these components, you will find it easier to organize and design exercise programs. This chapter also offers insights into other factors that affect adaptations and describes the changes and feelings you can expect from the various intensity levels of fitness. After reading this chapter, you will know how to monitor your training, making the whole process more enjoyable and more accurate.

The beauty of heart rate training is that it relies on a system (your cardiovascular system) that reflects your overall state of stress 24 hours a day, 365 days a year. It reflects when you're tired, overtrained, sick, cold, or hot and therefore can guide you in making changes to your plan. More important from an exercise point of view, it provides immediate and consistent feedback about your stress level, intensity level, and rate of adaptation in terms of overall fitness.

Because heart rate reveals how you are adapting to training, it is a valuable monitoring tool for exercise. Once you understand how to monitor and interpret your heart rate response to any given exercise scenario, and how to respond (i.e., rest, increase intensity, or decrease intensity), you will be able to optimize your fitness adaptations.

This chapter provides information to help you monitor, understand, and interpret your heart rate, thereby giving you the independence to individualize your workouts. But before we go into details, we have some important background information to cover.

Four Components of Physical Fitness

The four components of fitness—endurance, stamina, economy, and speed—are developed in phases. This is also their order of progression as you train. Figure 1.1, the basic model for training, shows these components schematically. Each develops at a specific intensity, and in the early stages of training is optimally developed within a very specific intensity range. Exercising above or below the intensity range will result in varied adaptations such as increased risk of injury, premature peaking, or staleness from overtraining, all of which result in poor performance. Each component has a zone with upper and lower limits. Heart rate is the simplest and most effective way to monitor intensity and therefore ensure training in the correct zone.

Endurance (phase I) is the ability to go from point A to point B no matter how much you have to slow down. In general, aerobic endurance is developed at heart rates of less than 75 percent of the maximum heart rate (percent MHR). Think of this phase of conditioning as getting into shape. If you wish to simply stay healthy, this is as hard as you have to work. Long, slow distances (LSD) are examples of endurance workouts.

Stamina (phase II) is the ability to go from point A to point B without slowing down. In general, stamina is developed in heart rate zones of 75 to 85 percent MHR. Consider this phase of conditioning as getting ready to race. The fitness emphasis in this phase is on preparing the cardiovascular and respiratory systems to work hard without overreaching. Steady-state workouts of 40 to 45 minutes are good examples of stamina workouts.

Economy (phase III) is the ability to go at race pace while using the least amount of oxygen and energy. In general, economy is developed in heart rate zones of 85 to 95 percent MHR. Think of this phase of conditioning as improving your racing fitness by adding more horsepower to your engine through workouts such as interval training, hill sprints, and fartlek running. (*Fartlek*, which literally means "speed play," is a Swedish system of conditioning that features frequent changes in speed.) Good examples of economy workouts are those at moderate to high intensity for continuous tempo paces, or interval workouts featuring longer repetitions.

Speed (phase IV) is the ability to go at top speeds for short periods of time and to stay relaxed while tolerating increasing levels of lactic acid in the muscle tissue. In general, speed is developed in heart rate zones of 95 to 100 percent MHR. The power training in this phase also will bring about final improvements in strength, flexibility, and coordination. Interval workouts of shorter, faster, and maximum-intensity repeats with long and full recoveries are the best examples of speed workouts.

These are not dictionary or laboratory terms, but are commonly used in the popular literature when discussing exercise and fitness. They are useful for identifying the heart rate ranges so you can safely progress up the training triangle all the way to championship shape, depending on your goal.

We start by identifying these concepts because they tie in well with the concept of oxygen usage, which, of course, is conveniently estimated (albeit indirectly) by your heart rate. When working on endurance, you will exercise in your aerobic effort zone. If you are focusing on improving speed, you will train in your anaerobic effort zone. Figure 1.1 is our version of the classic training triangle and offers a graphic representation of this approach.

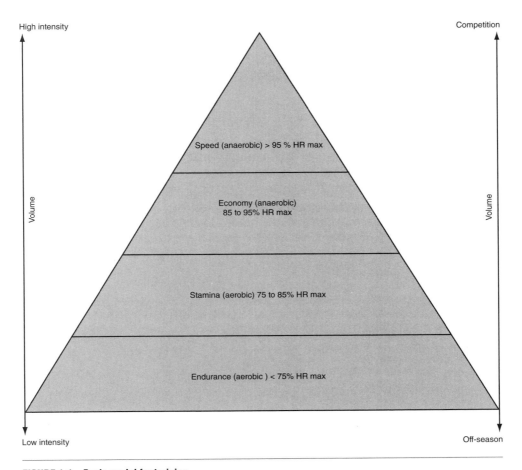

FIGURE 1.1   **Basic model for training.**

Activities in the lower, easier zone result in specific physiological and biomechanical adaptations, whereas those in the upper, harder zone have their own important biochemical and neurological adaptations. Developing speed requires fairly sophisticated training methods at even narrower effort zones within the anaerobic section of the triangle. These will be discussed in more detail in later chapters.

Table 1.1 illustrates another graphic way to express much of what we have covered so far and will talk about in later chapters.

Consider the categories in table 1.1 with a fair degree of open-mindedness because the zones range as wide as 10 to 15 percent. The reason for this is that, in our experience, people generally run more comfortably at higher heart rates than they bike, row, or swim. While running in your endurance zone, you might be closer to the 70 to 75 percent mark; whereas when swimming, you may be close to the 60 to 65 percent mark. When you become well trained, you will be able to perform more comfortably toward the upper level, which is the way we'd expect you to progress. An additional point about your maximum heart rate numbers: they will be different for each activity. Therefore, you will need a true maximum heart rate for each activity, especially if you're a triathlete. We will talk more about this in later chapters.

Personal Considerations

Essentially, all people are the same, made from the same parts. However, important differences, such as training objectives, affect our responses and adaptations.

Do you want to improve your cardiovascular health and control your weight? If so, then we suggest that you exercise frequently and extensively at the very low levels of aerobic endurance effort, but don't expect dramatic short-term gains. You need to make exercise a lifestyle.

Does simply participating (but not really competing) in a 10K road race with the goal of just finishing with a smile seem like a good way to enjoy some social recreation? If so, then for several months to a year, patiently increase

TABLE 1.1 Heart Rate Phases

HR zone	Effort index	Effort level	Pace	Fuel source	Fuel system	Fitness component
I	60–75%	Easy (EZ)	Slow	Primarily fats	Aerobic	Endurance
II	75–85%	Moderate (MO)	Moderate	Mix carbs and fats	Mix of aerobic and anaerobic	Stamina
III	85–95%	Difficult (FA)	Fast	Primarily carbs	Anaerobic	Economy
IV	95–100%	Very hard (VF)	Sprint	All carbs	ATP-PC	Speed

the volume of your endurance training, but substitute a couple days of training in the stamina zone of the triangle.

Do you want to compete and work hard at improving and setting personal records (PRs)? If so, you will need to add at least a day per week of high-intensity, anaerobic economy or speed workouts at the very difficult and mentally challenging level.

The preceding are some general ideas to get you thinking about your training goals. Your reasons will affect your target heart rate choices. Your responses and adaptations, however, also will be affected by something else: your genetic makeup.

Everyone understands that an easy effort results in a low heart rate and a harder effort raises it. Although this is true

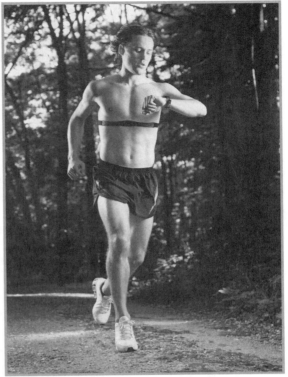

Valentin Casarsa

Your personal training goals and genetics will affect your responses to heart rate training.

for the most part, the relationship is not uniformly predictable especially in terms of absolute numbers. What this means is that two people exercising at the same absolute heart rate (145 beats per minute [bpm], for example) may have very different comfort levels. Genetic differences such as the composition of fast- and slow-twitch muscle fibers can result in puzzling heart rate responses. Fast-twitch fibers (think sprinters) have different oxygen consumption rates than slow-twitch fibers do (think marathoners). Another factor that can result in widely different heart rates in two people of similar ability and fitness level is the anatomy and size of the heart. These differences may result in heart rates that differ from 35 to 70 bpm in people running at the same pace.

Target heart rates are a lot like salaries—it's best not to discuss them. Having a higher heart rate than someone else does not mean that you are less fit.

One last genetic issue to point out is significant but far less remarkable—the difference in the heart size of males and females. This difference is revealed by the average resting heart rates of 72 bpm for men versus 84 bpm for women. This book will help you monitor your training by showing you how to measure your cardiac response to *your* program designed around *your* specific goals.

Rate of Perceived Exertion: Your Backup System

Individualizing workouts assumes that you understand the difference between hard and easy effort. (The former makes you grimace and gasp for air, whereas the latter allows you to laugh and talk all the way home.) Each of us can make subjective distinctions between hard and easy tasks. Before telemetric heart rate monitors made counting pulses so convenient, the rate of perceived exertion (RPE), as illustrated by the Borg Scale, was the standard for using one's own capacity for subjective measurement of hard and easy exercise effort. Dr. Borg's 15-point scale could be used, for example, to describe how average people might feel as they progressed from walking a mile to trying to run it in 4 minutes. The scale describes resting or walking as a very, very light effort, whereas exhaustion is described as beyond very, very hard. In addition, the Borg Scale also introduced a value system of points ranging from 6 (resting) to 20 (exhaustion). In short, Borg tried to correlate quantitative measures with his qualitative system. (Chapter 2 has more information on, and a complete chart of, the Borg Scale.)

Although the Borg Scale is useful, it is an arbitrary system because it offers no objective way to measure exertion. For the competitive athlete, a heart rate monitor is a better way to quantify those measurements. This book expands Borg's vocabulary to help you match your target heart rate to your perception of effort and, in the cases of running, rowing, swimming, and biking, to help you correlate your heart rate and perception of effort with your pace.

Probably the most important reason for individualizing training is the fact that people have different workout objectives. What exactly, as a percentage of your maximum, are your target heart rate zones? The need to calculate these zones is the challenge that brought us to share our collective wisdom with you. So, there are plenty of reasons for using the information in this book to help you use your heart rate monitor intelligently. Your body is not like anyone else's, so why work out like anyone else? Whatever your unique genetic gifts, current level of fitness, or goals are, this book will help you determine your target heart rates and individualize your training.

A quick word of caution: Not everyone will benefit from training with heart rate. By far the best applications are in endurance sports that require a somewhat steady pace for a period of time, usually in excess of 20 minutes. If you participate in team sports (soccer, rugby, football, lacrosse) and other nonaerobic settings such as wrestling, weightlifting, or boxing, be careful about using heart rate to train. Because of the start-and-stop nature of these sports, the use of heart rate to monitor intensity is somewhat limited; it really provides more information about energy expenditure and recovery than overall intensity. However, this doesn't mean that you cannot use heart rate if you participate in these sports; you can. Like aerobic athletes, you can use heart rate to monitor your training status and intensity during the aerobic training portion of your conditioning program or with interval training (a conditioning system that consists of repeated efforts over a time shorter than the length of the competition and done at fairly high intensities of 85 to 95 percent MHR), during which recovery heart rates are very valuable. It is also a useful recovery tool.

Using heart rate during higher-intensity anaerobic activity involves other, more complex physiological responses. Toward the end of the book, we provide more advice for using heart rate in the nonaerobic setting, but for now our focus is really on the typical endurance athlete—the runner, cyclist, rower, cross-country skier, triathlete, and so on.

What Heart Rate Reveals

Heart rate provides a lot of information, but you must have reliable data to interpret it correctly. Accurate data will allow you to evaluate your own responses, adaptations, energy expenditure, training programs, and a lot more. The take-home message for this section is that you are embarking on a quest for knowledge that is highly individualized and therefore likely to yield the results you want. Here is the possible information you can get from heart rate monitoring provided you have the right monitor and good data recording:

- Correct intensity for aerobic system development
- Correct intensity for anaerobic system development
- Correct durations for time spent in appropriate training zones
- Appropriate recovery periods during interval training
- Appropriate recovery periods between exercise sessions
- Effective evaluation of adaptations to training programs
- Early warning signs of overtraining
- Early indications of heat stress
- Early indications of energy depletion
- Race pace strategy for longer competitions

This list should convince you that heart rate training is indeed worthwhile (and these are only some of the benefits!).

Understanding Heart Rate

The simple beauty of monitoring heart rate is that it is based on your own heart's capacity and nobody else's. As you train and stress yourself, you can monitor your adaptations via heart rate. Your heart rate monitor is like an instant feedback machine, telling you whether you are training too hard or too easy, have recovered appropriately from a previous workout, have overtrained from a series of workouts, and are responding the right way to your training program.

The heart is a muscle, and it responds in much the same way as any other muscle by getting bigger and stronger as you work out. When you are not working out, the heart continues to pump blood into your muscles to feed their repair and recovery. That's why heart rate can inform you indirectly about the state of recovery of your muscles. If you still have microtears or are replacing fuel, your metabolism will be elevated and your heart rate will reflect that by being slightly higher. That's why monitoring and recording your heart rate each morning when you wake up will give you an idea of whether you're still under a condition of repair from a previous workout.

There are several important numbers with heart rate. Two important ones are your resting heart rate and your maximum heart rate. Maximum heart rate is the fastest, highest number of times the heart can beat in a minute. Resting heart rate is the heart beat at rest at its lowest, slowest number per minute (normally taken when you wake up in the morning).

Maximum heart rate doesn't really change as a result of training, but all your training zones are calculated from that number. Therefore, you need an accurate maximum heart rate (see the section on calculating maximum heart rate). Resting heart rate, on the other hand, does change with training and generally decreases with increasing fitness. At times, resting heart rate can increase, which usually indicates fatigue, overtraining, or sickness. Charting your resting heart rate can help identify these conditions fairly early.

Take a look at the resting heart rate response of a runner over a one-month period depicted in figure 1.2. Notice what happens on the days following a

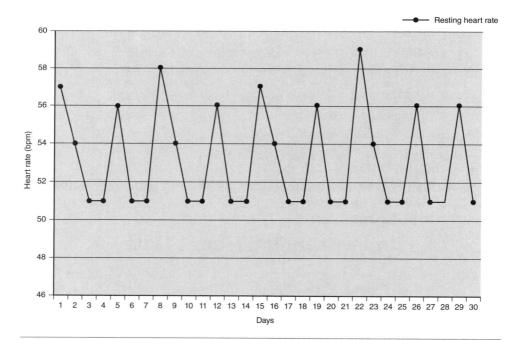

FIGURE 1.2 **Morning resting heart rate over a period of 30 days. Harder workouts occurred on the day before each spike.**

high-intensity sprint workout or a long run. Each time the athlete performed a hard session or a long run, the resting heart rate was elevated on the following day. This information is useful because it can help the athlete adjust his workouts when he is not fully recovered and possibly prevent overtraining and injury. This is an example of how heart rate monitoring can help plan recovery, but it is equally useful in determining exercise intensity.

Depending on the intensity of the exercise you're doing, you'll get a different adaptation throughout your body. We will simplify this by noting that easier exercise causes cardiovascular (aerobic) changes and harder exercise causes biochemical (anaerobic) changes. Both are necessary for good performance, and too much or too little of either will cause unwarranted adaptations. Your heart rate can help you determine the intensity of your training, thereby keeping you in the desired training zones. We'll talk more about calculating target zones in chapter 2.

Intensity Relationship of Heart Rate and Oxygen Consumption

Our discussion so far has focused on heart rate. However, oxygen uptake, a close cousin of heart rate, is often mentioned in the popular literature. Experts seem to contradict each other or, at the very least, confuse readers as they recommend that training take place at various percentages of either of these physical capacities. Furthermore, oxygen uptake capacity is abbreviated different ways, sometimes as $\dot{V}O_2$ or O_2 uptake. At any rate, $\dot{V}O_2$ refers to the volume of oxygen consumed, and $\dot{V}O_2$max refers to the greatest amount of oxygen someone can consume, which usually occurs at maximum exercise intensity. In general, the fitter you are, the higher your $\dot{V}O_2$max will be. Both heart rate and $\dot{V}O_2$ are ways to measure how hard (intensely) someone is working. Heart rate response is simply a measure of how hard the cardiovascular system is working to distribute oxygen, whereas $\dot{V}O_2$ measures include heart rate and the work of the respiratory system's and muscular system's use of oxygen.

During aerobic exercise, both heart rate and $\dot{V}O_2$ increase as intensity increases. However, the patterns of response for both variables are different. In science, terms such as *linear* and *nonlinear* are used to describe relationships between two variables. The term *linear* basically means that as one variable increases, the other variable increases in proportion to the change in the first variable. If one variable changes and the other changes but not in proportion, that is described as *nonlinear*.

Although both heart rate and $\dot{V}O_2$ increase in response to increasing intensity, their responses are not entirely linear. For example, at lower exercise intensities both variables increase in a similar manner, but at higher intensities the heart rate response levels off while the $\dot{V}O_2$ response continues to climb. This does not detract in any way from the value of the information but merely serves to show that responses do vary.

Another important difference in response patterns is that we see a dramatic and rapid increase in heart rate at the start of exercise regardless of the intensity. Someone who begins to jog slowly may see a 25- to 40-beat increase in heart rate right away that could go, for example, from 75 to 110 bpm. This heart rate will settle and may even decrease slightly after 5 to 10 minutes and eventually even out at 105 bpm. On the other hand, $\dot{V}O_2$ responds very slowly at the start of exercise, and we may see only a small change within 5 to 7 minutes that continues at a slow, steady pace even with abrupt changes in intensity. Heart rate will continue to respond abruptly at the lower intensities and then smooth out and change more slowly at the higher intensities. It is important to understand this relationship because it can help explain aspects of performance such as warm-up and recovery. Let's look at the overall relationship of heart rate, $\dot{V}O_2$, and intensity in a little more detail.

The relationship between heart rate and intensity is convenient. Although $\dot{V}O_2$max is considered the gold standard for measuring intensity and work capacity, its measurement is not easily available to the average athlete. This measurement needs to be done in a laboratory and can be expensive. But, if we can demonstrate a relationship between heart rate and $\dot{V}O_2$, we can use the more convenient measure of heart rate to monitor training sessions anywhere.

Table 1.2 shows what percentage of maximum heart rate you are working at based on your percentage of maximum oxygen uptake. For example, when you are working at 65 percent MHR, you are working at approximately 48 percent of $\dot{V}O_2$max. Remember, these numbers are not absolute; they represent an approximation of where you'll be at a certain heart rate and $\dot{V}O_2$. These numbers do vary a little more around the 70 percent mark, and for

TABLE 1.2 Percent MHR—$\dot{V}O_2$max Conversion Chart

Percent MHR	Corresponding percent $\dot{V}O_2$max	Training adaptation
50%	~22%	Minimal for trained athletes
55	~28	
60	~42	Phase I: Endurance
65	~48	
70	~52	
75	~60	Phase II: Stamina
80	~70	
85	~78	Phase III: Economy
90	~85	
95–100	~93	Phase IV: Speed

that reason, we need to use a range to ensure accuracy. In either situation, exercise slightly above or slightly below 75 percent still represents an easy to comfortable workload.

To further clarify the relationship between heart rate and $\dot{V}O_2$, let's consider some data from the Human Performance Laboratory at the University of Vermont. Tables 1.3 and 1.4 show recorded data from two subjects. One subject performed on a treadmill; and the other, on a bike. Both were fairly well-trained athletes.

TABLE 1.3 Data for a 19-Year-Old Female Cross-Country Skier*

Time (min)	Work rate (mph, % grade)	Heart rate (bpm)	$\dot{V}O_2$ (ml/kg/min)
0:30	5, 0%	51	4.1
1:00	5, 0%	93	11.3
1:30	5, 0%	107	19.9
2:00	5, 0%	116	29.5
2:30	5, 0%	115	29.7
3:00	6, 0%	117	29.5
3:30	6, 0%	120	29.1
4:00	6, 0%	118	28.5
4:30	6, 0%	126	30.3
5:00	7, 0%	128	31.7
5:30	7, 0%	132	31.9
6:00	7, 0%	137	36.0
6:30	7, 0%	142	34.9
7:00	7.5, 0%	144	38.0
7:30	7.5, 0%	150	37.7
8:00	7.5, 0%	153	37.7
8:30	7.5, 0%	154	40.3
9:00	8.0, 0%	156	39.7
9:30	8.0, 0%	159	42.6
10:00	8.0, 0%	162	42.7
10:30	8.0, 0%	163	45.0
11:00	8.5, 0%	163	41.6
11:30	8.5, 0%	166	45.9
12:00	8.5, 0%	167	47.3
12:30	8.5, 0%	171	45.9

(continued)

TABLE 1.3 *(continued)*

Time (min)	Work rate (mph, % grade)	Heart rate (bpm)	$\dot{V}O_2$ (ml/kg/min)
13:00	8.5, 2%	173	46.4
13:30	8.5, 2%	171	47.5
14:00	8.5, 2%	173	48.3
14:30	8.5, 2%	174	50.7
15:00	8.5, 4%	173	51.6
15:30	8.5, 4%	176	54.8
16:00	8.5, 4%	180	54.8
16:30	8.5, 4%	183	54.7
17:00	8.5, 4%	183	58.2
17:30	8.5, 4%	182	58.1
18:00	8.5, 6%	182	59.6
18:30	8.5, 6%	183	61.2
19:00	8.5, 6%	183	64.2

*Test subject performed on a treadmill.
*Anaerobic threshold: 171 bpm; max $\dot{V}O_2$: 64.2 ml/kg/min; MHR: 183.

TABLE 1.4 Data for a 45-Year-Old Male Cyclist*

Time (min)	Work rate (watts)	Heart rate (bpm)	$\dot{V}O_2$ (ml/kg/min)
0:30	120	110	3.4
1:00	120	109	7.0
1:30	120	105	24.0
2:00	120	104	25.0
2:30	120	100	26.1
3:00	180	102	22.3
3:30	180	109	27.3
4:00	180	113	28.1
4:30	180	114	31.8
5:00	240	115	32.3
5:30	240	118	33.2
6:00	240	127	36.8
6:30	240	130	41.6
7:00	280	134	42.8
7:30	280	139	42.4

Time (min)	Work rate (watts)	Heart rate (bpm)	$\dot{V}O_2$ (ml/kg/min)
8:00	280	141	45.7
8:30	280	142	47.3
9:00	320	145	48.0
9:30	320	149	50.4
10:00	320	152	53.0
10:30	320	156	51.5
11:00	360	156	57.9
11:30	360	159	56.1
12:00	360	163	59.5
12:30	360	164	58.4
13:00	400	167	62.2
13:30	400	169	62.8
14:00	400	172	64.8
14:30	400	173	67.0
15:00	410	173	66.0
15:30	410	175	68.3
16:00	410	177	67.2

*Test subject performed on a bicycle.
*Anaerobic threshold: 152 bpm; max $\dot{V}O_2$: 68.3 ml/kg/min; MHR: 177 bpm.

The tables note data for work rate, $\dot{V}O_2$max (ml/kg/min), and heart rate (bpm). The other data of importance for both subjects is anaerobic threshold, which is noted in the footnotes. Pay attention to the anaerobic threshold data because we can use these as a reference point to demonstrate the relationships between heart rate and $\dot{V}O_2$. Anaerobic threshold will be discussed in greater detail in chapter 6. For now, note that anaerobic threshold is the point at which you see heart rate creep up a little faster. It also is the point at which you increase your anaerobic metabolism, which results in faster breathing, a higher heart rate, and less talking.

Using heart rate calculations, you will see that subject 1 has an anaerobic threshold that occurs at 92 percent MHR but only 70 percent of $\dot{V}O_2$max. For subject 2, the heart rate at anaerobic threshold occurs at 86 percent MHR but only 77 percent of $\dot{V}O_2$max. In other words, intensities will always be lower when calculated as a function of $\dot{V}O_2$max. The pattern of response also is different between the two variables, and this partially explains the different percentages. $\dot{V}O_2$max has a pretty linear relationship with work intensity, whereas heart rate is linear only up to 75 to 80 percent intensity. Then it flattens out and is nonlinear as you get closer to maximum (see figure 1.3).

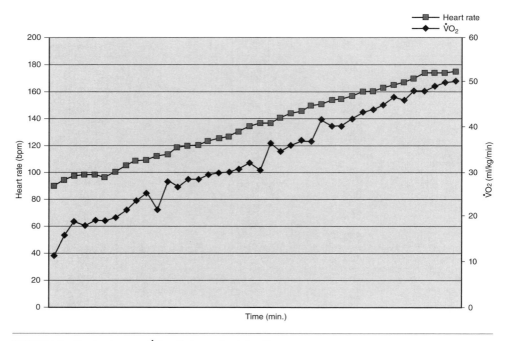

FIGURE 1.3 **Heart rate versus V̇O₂ with increasing intensity.**

Understanding this relationship is important because heart rate is a more reliable indicator of changes in fitness at any given workload. $\dot{V}O_2$, on the other hand, is a better indicator of energy expenditure because energy expenditure is directly related to $\dot{V}O_2$. This is important because heart rate response to a given workload will decrease with advancing fitness. $\dot{V}O_2$, or energy expenditure, actually will stay about the same for a given workload unless the subject loses weight.

Figure 1.4 illustrates the fitness testing of a 40-year-old male subject before and after a brief training program. (These data are also presented in table 1.5.) The subject was tested after three months of training. Even though his body weight didn't change much (he lost 4 pounds, or 1.8 kilograms), his heart rate decreased over time but his $\dot{V}O_2$ stayed pretty much the same at all sub-maximum values; then increased at maximum over time, showing improved fitness. Interestingly, maximum heart rate was the same as pretraining data even though the ending work rate was substantially higher.

This is exactly the outcome you would like to have after a period of training—lower heart rate at a fixed workload, same $\dot{V}O_2$max at a fixed workload, but the $\dot{V}O_2$max is a lower percentage of maximum capacity because maximum capacity has increased. (Improved skill levels also can contribute to the improvement of oxygen uptake capacity.) Both of these outcomes have to do with efficiency. The $\dot{V}O_2$max increases because of an increased cardiorespiratory network in heart, lung, and skeletal muscle; improved oxygen extraction; and improved fat metabolism. The heart rate at the fixed

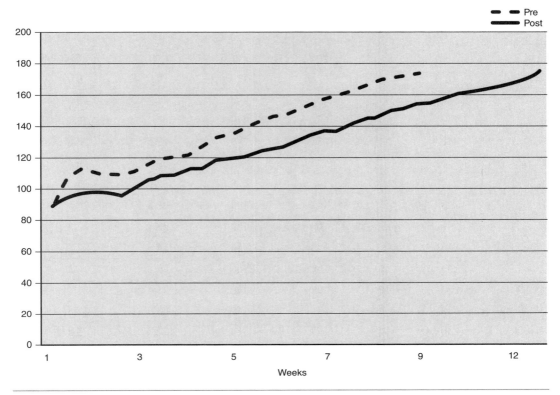

FIGURE 1.4 Heart data for a 40-year-old male before and after 12 weeks of easy baseline training. Data were collected on a bicycle in response to the same workload.

TABLE 1.5 Pre- and Posttraining Data for a 40-Year-Old Male Cyclist*

Time (min)	Work rate (watts)	Heart rate (bpm)		$\dot{V}O_2$ (ml/kg/min)	
		Pretraining	Posttraining	Pretraining	Posttraining
0:30	105	89	90	12.3	11.4
1:00	105	107	94	18.0	16.0
1:30	105	113	97	20.6	19.0
2:00	105	110	98	20.0	18.3
2:30	105	109	98	19.1	19.3
3:00	140	109	96	19.9	19.0
3:30	140	111	100	19.6	19.9
4:00	140	115	105	21.4	21.5
4:30	140	119	108	24.0	23.5
5:00	175	120	109	23.2	25.2
5:30	175	121	112	23.2	21.6

(continued)

TABLE 1.5 *(continued)*

Time (min)	Work rate (watts)	Heart rate (bpm)		$\dot{V}O_2$ (ml/kg/min)	
		Pretraining	Posttraining	Pretraining	Posttraining
6:00	175	127	113	26.6	28.0
6:30	175	132	118	27.1	26.6
7:00	210	134	119	28.1	28.4
7:30	210	137	120	29.0	28.3
8:00	210	141	123	30.3	29.4
8:30	210	145	125	32.0	31.7
9:00	245	147	126	32.3	31.1
9:30	245	150	130	33.3	32.6
10:00	245	153	134	34.0	33.0
10:30	245	156	136	35.2	34.5
11:00	280	158	136	37.4	36.4
11:30	280	161	140	38.5	37.6
12:00	280	164	143	39.0	39.0
12:30	280	167	145	41.5	40.1
13:00	315	169	149	41.4	41.8
13:30	315	171	150	43.4	42.6
14:00	315	173	153	43.1	43.2
14:30	315		154		43.2
15:00	350		156		44.7
15:30	350		159		44.2
16:00	350		160		45.9
16:30	350		162		45.9
17:00	385		164		46.5
17:30	385		166		47.0
18:00	385		169		48.1
18:30	385		173		48.9

*Test subject performed on a stationary bicycle.

load decreases because the heart muscle is now stronger and can move more blood with each beat. The technical term for this is *improved stroke volume.* Later in the book we revisit these data by expanding them to look at power production at a given heart rate and how this can be used to improve fitness.

Energy Expenditure Relationship Between Heart Rate and $\dot{V}O_2$

So far we have looked at the relationship between heart rate and intensity, the relationship between percent MHR and percent $\dot{V}O_2$max, and how these variables can change with appropriate training over time. An important take-home point is that there is a subtle difference in the response of both heart rate and $\dot{V}O_2$. As mentioned previously, heart rate is linear only up to about 90 to 95 percent MHR, and then it really smoothes out and changes little in response to increasing workload. On the other hand, $\dot{V}O_2$ continues to increase fairly steadily all the way until maximum capacity. Figure 1.3 (page 16) shows the HR–$\dot{V}O_2$ relationship to a maximum exercise test. If you take a close look at the data, you'll see that heart rate actually reaches maximum before $\dot{V}O_2$ does. This means that you can actually increase intensity and energy expenditure at maximum heart rate but not $\dot{V}O_2$max.

As intensity increases, so does energy expenditure, and $\dot{V}O_2$ reflects energy expenditure better than heart rate does. When we test subjects in the lab, we always determine energy expenditure from the oxygen consumption rates or O_2 uptake. To do this, we need to understand the basic relationship between energy expenditure (calories burned) and $\dot{V}O_2$. When people get a $\dot{V}O_2$ test, their scores are normally reported in milliliters of oxygen per kilogram of body weight per min (ml/kg/min). However, these data are actually recorded in liters per minute (L/min) and then converted to milliliters afterward. Consider this example of a 60-kilogram runner:

Runner weight: 60 kg

$\dot{V}O_2$max in L/min: 4.0 L/min

$\dot{V}O_2$max in ml/kg/min: 4.0 L $\times$ 1,000 = 4,000 ml

$$4,000 \text{ ml} / 60 \text{ kg} = 66.6 \text{ ml/kg/min}$$

The question is, How much energy expenditure is taking place at this level? To answer this question, you need to remember the following relationship: 1 L oxygen = 5 cal. Therefore, a runner consuming 4.0 L/min (or 66 ml/kg/min) is burning approximately 20 calories per minute. Now we can calculate the energy expenditure for any athlete in any sport at any intensity with some basic data. But more important, you can see that energy expenditure is a function of oxygen consumption and not necessarily of heart rate because the heart rate response to exercise changes as a function of many factors (which we'll discuss in chapter 3), whereas $\dot{V}O_2$ actually tends to stay the same at rest or at any given workload.

Any treadmill or stationary bike these days can calculate calories burned. When you exercise, you are basically moving a given load (your body weight) at a given speed or over a distance, or overcoming a load, such as the resistance on a bike. This provides a few known variables, basically loads or forces and distances. Using this information, we can calculate how much oxygen is needed to perform the workload. From there, we apply our 1 L oxygen = 5 cal calculation to get energy expenditure.

When you get on a treadmill, the system asks for your weight. From there, it uses the speed and grade you select to calculate the rest. A stationary bike doesn't need your body weight. Instead, it uses the selected level of resistance as the weight. As you get fitter, the $\dot{V}O_2$ requirement doesn't change because the load stays the same, but your heart rate should decrease in response to the same load. This is another good way to use heart rate to evaluate fitness response to a given workload. Now you can select a workout with the goal of burning a certain number of calories and even take it outside.

By now you're well on your way to understanding the relationships among intensity, heart rate, and $\dot{V}O_2$ and can calculate anaerobic threshold and heart rate changes at a given pace to changes in fitness over time, among other things. The coming chapters will add to your knowledge of how and why to use heart rate to guide your training program.

CHAPTER 2

Evaluating and Customizing Your Zones

This chapter addresses what the heart rate numbers should look like depending on your chosen intensity. We also discuss calculating both maximum heart rate (MHR) and target heart rate zone properly. As we do this, we identify sources of error in the measurements so you'll know right away if there's a problem. Finally, we discuss how the numbers should change as you progress with your exercise program. Most important, you'll understand how to manipulate your training times and intensities by using heart rate to ensure that you optimize your training and adaptations. We've included additional information about the heart rate response and distribution of the population in general to give you a bigger overall picture. However, we start with the basics—getting used to the heart rate monitor and learning what the numbers mean.

Facts and Myths About Heart Rate Numbers

What do heart rate numbers mean? Before interpreting the numbers, we'd like to share our experience in understanding heart rate responses to exercise. This is one of the most important benefits of this book because this information is seldom included in the instruction manuals that come with heart rate monitors. Knowing some basic truths and common misunderstandings can help you avoid getting false feedback from your monitor. Take the following true/false quiz to see how well you understand heart rate:

1. The popular formula of subtracting your age from 220 bpm for predicting MHR is reliable for everyone.
2. Treadmill or bike testing for MHR is not a learned skill and takes no experience.
3. Treadmill or bike cardiac stress tests administered in physicians' offices often fall far short of revealing actual true MHR.
4. A heart rate number is a heart rate number. In other words, once you've got a heart rate training zone for any sport, you can apply it across a range of sports.

All in all, what you see on a heart rate monitor will be reliable and valid. But too many people who have spent money on monitors bury them in the back of their sock drawers and are not using them because they have become frustrated by irrational numbers. So, let's see how you did on the quiz.

Myth 1: Predicting Maximum Heart Rate

The idea that anyone can subtract his or her age from 220 bpm to predict a reliable MHR is a myth. Here's a real-life example from Bob Johnson, who has an exceptional heart. When he bought a monitor at age 55, he had no idea that his MHR was way above predicted average. By using the age-adjusted formula suggested in the instructions that came with the monitor, he calculated his MHR to be 165. Using the standard target HR zone of 60 to 70 percent for an easy aerobic workout, he set his receiver to beep when he was outside the zone of 99 to 115 bpm. Bob went out for a jog but within minutes was exceeding 115 bpm. He slowed down to keep the alarm from sounding. In another few minutes, he was reduced to walking and then to a crawl to keep his monitor quiet. This was not the monitor's fault. It was merely doing its job by warning him that he was out of his target zone. Bob knew that he was not in bad shape for his age, but this was shocking. After a few more workouts, Bob's puzzlement over his new purchase was growing into a good case of frustration.

What went wrong? Bob didn't realize that he had a smaller-than-average heart and that it could compensate by being able to reach a much higher MHR. In fact, his actual MHR turned out to be an even 200 bpm, 35 beats higher than predicted by the conventional formula.

So what's the story? Let's start with this fact: The average MHR of a brand new baby, who has a heart the size of a walnut, is 220 bpm. And we know that as a person grows up, the heart also grows bigger. At adulthood, the heart is about the size of the person's fist. Naturally, it has more capacity for holding blood in its chambers. This means that more blood is pumped with each stroke (greater stroke volume), and hence, fewer beats are required. By age 20, growth of the heart brings the average MHR down to about 195 bpm. From that age, the aging process causes a further decline at the convenient rate of about a beat per year. This explains the logic of the formula: 220 minus age equals predicted MHR.

Now here is the key to understanding why Bob could hit 200 at age 55. Maximum heart rates are naturally spread across the standard distribution of a bell-shaped curve. As with intelligence, there is a wide range from one end of the curve to the other for people of the same age. This distribution means only that those at the mean can reliably predict MHR by using the age-adjusted formulas. Depending on where you fall on the curve, your MHR may be as high as 36 bpm above or below what the formula predicts.

Trust us on this one. Way before telemetric heart rate monitors, when we used our fingers to palpate carotid arteries (the jugular vein in the neck), we counted maximum heart rates as high as 200 and as low as 140 bpm for 50-year-olds. People with high maximum heart rates simply have smaller but much quicker hearts. Some young adults whose hearts are as big as grapefruits have maximum heart rates of 140 to 160 bpm at truly drop-dead levels of fatigue, and this is normal. Admittedly, these examples are few and far between, but they do exist, and maybe you're one of them. The bottom line: You need an accurate measure of maximum heart rate.

Myth 2: Enduring Fitness Testing

It's true that someone not experienced with exhaustive levels of athletic effort might not do well on a first max treadmill stress test. So the idea that treadmill or bike testing for MHR is not a learned skill and takes no experience is a myth.

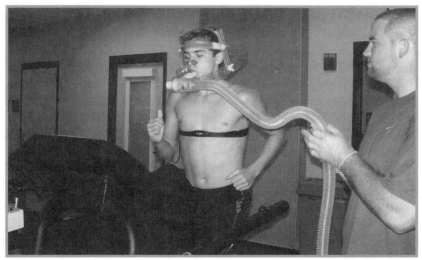

Declan Connolly

Even an endurance fitness test in a clinical setting may not accurately reveal true maximum heart rate. An athlete has to push himself until his heart rate plateaus, which is beyond what many people can endure.

People often bail out long before they reach their true maximum values because they don't know how to endure the pain of full fatigue or they simply are unfamiliar with this level of effort and are very uncomfortable with it. True MHR is not reached until the beats per minute plateau and refuse to rise any higher no matter how much harder, faster, or longer the subject moves. Most rookies have to survive several close brushes with exhaustion before they realize how hard they can push themselves and what levels of fatigue they can endure and live to tell about. If you have suspicions about your MHR, keep trying.

Myth 3: Getting a Real Maximum Effort

Doctors usually don't like to stand around watching patients perform heroic feats of athletic endurance during exercise stress tests. Because doctors are in the business of detecting hidden heart disease, treadmill or bike cardiac stress tests administered in a physician's office are usually submaximal and don't reveal true MHR. Symptoms of coronary artery problems usually surface once the subject reaches or slightly exceeds anaerobic threshold (AT). Despite the fact that the anaerobic threshold is fitness dependent and can be experienced by unfit folks at very low percentages of MHR, it is expected by most doctors to be about 85 percent MHR. So once the effort level is achieved, often the test is ended with the subject far short of the real MHR. Furthermore, most physicians are not well educated in exercise physiology and often naively use the age-adjusted formula for predicting that target in the first place. (See the first myth for why this is not a good idea.) If you are still suspicious about your real MHR, keep reading.

Myth 4: Applying Heart Rate Responses Across Exercise Modes

Heart rate responses vary depending on work rate across exercise modes. What this means is that a 60 percent MHR while running can feel completely different than a 60 percent MHR while cycling or swimming. Triathletes know this only too well. Heart rate varies as a function of many variables; one is the number of active muscle contractions and whether you are carrying your weight, as in running, pushing it, as in cycling, or pulling it, in a supported environment as in swimming. Therefore, multisport athletes should have different heart rate values for different activities. Your familiarity with an activity and the specificity of the activity affect your heart rate response.

Determining Maximum Heart Rate

As you contemplate determining your true maximum heart rate, think back to the information presented for myth 1 (page 22). Make sure you have accurate data based on you in your chosen activity. The sport-specific chapters provide more relevant information on this topic, but we want to emphasize here how important it is to have this information.

This section presents some protocols for self-testing in running. (The protocols for swimming, cycling, rowing, and cross-country skiing are in those specific chapters.)

Not knowing your own MHR is the first error. If you don't know your actual MHR, you could be in exactly the same shape, have exactly the same running ability, and be running the same pace as your training partner while your respective heart rates are as much as 72 beats apart in extreme cases. Remember what we said about comparing heart rates: Don't do it. Furthermore, be skeptical when using a monitor for the first time if the numbers you've calculated from the predicted max formula don't seem to make sense. Take a treadmill stress test supervised by a physiologist or physician who promises to take you to your maximum. Obviously, a testing facility is the safest and most effective place to be tested for your MHR. Some universities offer these services, as do higher-end sport clubs, sports medicine clinics, and even some private practitioners. Cost ranges from $100 to $350.

Choose where you get tested carefully. There is a lot of room for interpretation and measurement error depending on the skill of the technician. Look for certified technicians and exercise physiologists and not a self-professed fitness enthusiast who took a weekend course and bought some equipment. Simple testing protocols, such as the running test described here, are useful for most people but may not tell the whole story, depending on your level of fitness, skill, and mode of activity. If you suspect your numbers aren't right, try the tests in the programming chapters. Before undergoing any testing, be sure to get the okay from your doctor.

Sample Running Test for MHR

1. Find a running track or a small and gradual incline that goes for about 400 to 600 meters. Put on your heart rate monitor.
2. Do a good 0.5- to 1-mile warm-up (0.8 to 1.6 km).
3. Perform one lap or one incline lap as fast as you can. Check your heart rate at the end of the lap.
4. Take a 2-minute recovery walk or run, and then repeat the run. Again, check your heart rate when you finish.
5. Take a 2-minute recovery, and repeat the run again. Again, check your heart rate when you finish. Your heart rate at the end of this third trial will be a pretty good indicator of your maximum heart rate.

Calculating Target Heart Rate or Heart Rate Training Zones

The level of stimulus to your organs affects their rate of adaptation. As you might expect, lower-intensity activity has a different effect than higher-intensity activity does. You have probably heard the terms *aerobic* and *anaerobic metabolism* or *aerobic* and *anaerobic energy systems.* Think of *aerobic* and *anaerobic* as synonymous with *low intensity* and *high intensity. Aerobic* means "with oxygen," as in "Let's talk while we jog." *Anaerobic* means the opposite (without oxygen), as in "We're going so hard that I'm too out of breath to talk now."

These terms have several implications for training. How effectively you develop these systems is of major importance in how you perform. For the most part, the information in this book targets the endurance, or aerobic, athlete. However, top-class endurance performances also depend heavily on anaerobic energy. If peak performances are your objective, it would be a fatal mistake to have a well-developed aerobic system without an appropriately developed anaerobic system. Conversely, it usually is a mistake to try anaerobic workouts without first developing a base of endurance from aerobic training.

You can also differentiate between aerobic and anaerobic work this way: Lower-intensity, aerobic work at heart rates lower than 75 percent MHR induces cardiovascular and body composition changes, whereas higher-intensity, anaerobic work at heart rates greater than 80 percent induces more neural, respiratory, and biochemical changes. Unfortunately, endurance athletes often pay too much attention to long, slow aerobic miles and not enough attention to the "bone crusher" anaerobic workouts, which is what the Kenyans call their high-intensity track workouts. We'll come back to these issues later in the book.

Because the right intensity ensures the right adaptations, you need to not only fully understand the reason for each target heart rate zone, but also trust the accuracy of the numbers on your monitor. To ensure that your workout meets its objective, and that the beats per minute on your monitor make sense, match them with a backup system. Of course, the preferable way to regulate intensity is to measure it objectively with your heart rate monitor. Measuring it subjectively may take some experience, but it is a practical and easily learned method. The Borg Scale of Perceived Exertion is the best subjective method.

There are several methods of calculating target heart rate zones. However, these are all predictions and can yield varying results. We include them here so you can see how much room for error there is when predicting. You can use these approaches, but we suggest that you get an actual measurement.

These are the more common calculation methods:

Equation 1: 220 − age (years) = MHR

Equation 2: 210 − [0.5 × age (years)] = MHR

Equation 3: Karvonen formula

The Karvonen formula uses 220 − age (years) for MHR, but it doesn't stop there. Here is the full formula:

220 − age (years) = MHR

MHR − resting heart rate (RHR) = heart rate reserve (HRR)

Intensity = % × HRR + RHR

In recent years there has been speculation that MHR varies between males and females. As science continues to explore this topic, there is a mixed consensus on which gender has the higher MHR. The following formulas are adjusted to accommodate this gender effect.

Equation 4 (males): 202 − [0.55 × age (years)]

Equation 5 (females): 216 − [1.09 × age (years)]

Note that age is the determining factor in all calculations. It is well established that MHR declines with increasing age, and age alone is pretty much the primary determining factor. However, like most physiological variables, there is a high degree of individual variation. Consider the following numbers based on calculating 70 to 80 percent training zones for a 40-year-old with a resting heart rate of 65 bpm using each method.

Equation 1

220 − 40 (age in years) = 180 bpm

180 bpm (MHR) × 0.7 (70%) = 126; 180 bpm × 0.8 (80%) = 144

Training zone = 126 to 144 bpm

Equation 2

210 − 20 [0.5 × 40 (age in years)] = 190 bpm

190 bpm (MHR) × 0.7 (70%) = 133; 190 bpm × 0.8 (80%) = 152

Training zone = 133 to 152 bpm

Equation 3

220 − 40 (age in years) = 180 bpm

180 bpm (MHR) − 65 bpm (RHR) = 115 bpm (HRR)

0.7 (70%) × 115 bpm (HRR) + 65 bpm (RHR) = 145.5 bpm

0.8 (80%) × 115 bpm + 65 bpm = 157

Training zone = 145 to 157 bpm

Equation 4

202 − [0.55 × 40 (age in yrs)] = 202 − 22 = 180 bpm

Training zone = 126 to 144 bpm

Equation 5

216 − [1.09 × 40 (age in yrs)] = 216 − 43.6 = 172.4 bpm

Training zone = 121 to 138 bpm

Using these simple figures alone, we have up to a 17 percent variation in the low-end exercise heart rate. For serious athletes, this is a huge difference that will yield considerable variations in training outcomes. This problem may be compounded if we are unsure about the correctness of any of these numbers.

Note that the major limitation in all calculations is the absence of a true measure of MHR. This is really what all athletes need individually and should determine periodically during their training phases. Multisport athletes should be measured for all sports because MHR varies according to activity modes. This measurement does not require sophisticated equipment but an accurately administered and progressive protocol that incrementally exhausts the athlete in 12 to 15 minutes. This often requires a little experience because if you fatigue too early or too late, you often don't get good data. Many facilities that offer these services do not understand proper methodology and consequently generate inaccurate data, much to the frustration of the client who then uses it for months without the desired adaptations. You'll need a heart rate monitor and the ability to record the MHR you achieve during the session. (Typically it occurs as you become exhausted.)

When we fitness test, we use a telemetry system that allows us to constantly monitor the response and also relate the heart rate response to wattage, speed, 500-meter splits, and so on. This number yields much greater accuracy than a traditional prediction equation does.

Also, you need to be aware that a small spike in MHR often follows the cessation of maximum exercise; this should not be considered a sustainable MHR. This is another common mistake.

Remember that different modes of exercise yield different responses. Running yields a higher MHR than cycling does for most people. However, trained cyclists and rowers have higher MHRs in their chosen sports than they have running. Therefore, rowers should perform this trial on rowing ergometers or on the water. Cyclists should perform the trial on bikes; and runners, on treadmills. Each athlete should have his or her own individually measured MHR.

Research data show variations in calculated heart rates quite nicely as a function of mode. They first showed the variation in MHR as a function of mode and also that running produced MHR numbers close to the 220 – age equation. The numbers generated on the treadmill were significantly different from the numbers generated using other exercise modes. The numbers generated during cycling were significantly less than predicted (on average 18 bpm) and varied from −35 bpm to +16 bpm. Cycling data were on average 96 percent of treadmill data. A meta-analysis by some authors suggested that age accounted for about 75 percent of MHR variability, but others have reported that age actually accounts for a lower percentage of the variability. On average, the heart rate variability from age-predicted MHR is ±10 to 12 bpm.

Using the data from our earlier calculated example, we now see that a 40-year-old using a prediction equation could exercise anywhere from 121 to 145 bpm and assume it was 70 percent MHR. This is a large variation and not altogether accurate. The take-home message is that many of us will have an MHR that varies significantly from the predicted values, and if we are using these equations, may be well off the mark. Therefore, a simple approach to increase accuracy and reliability is to measure your own MHR and then calculate your percentage of intensity using this real number.

Note: The determination of MHR requires a maximum effort and therefore presents a potentially dangerous situation for certain people. Consequently, qualified personnel should perform your testing.

Balancing Numbers With Common Sense

The fallback method of gauging the intensity levels of your workouts features the use of common sense in the form of perceived exertion. The perceived exertion scale was developed by scientist Gunnar Borg back in the early 1960s. Dr. Borg was actually more into psychosomatic research and was interested in developing a feeling scale that could in some way be quantified. He developed the Rating of Perceived Exertion (RPE) chart. The original scale ran from 6 to 20 with verbal cues describing perceived exertion on the odd numbers. The scale has undergone several editions since the early work of Dr. Borg.

The scale of 6 to 20 actually describes the range of adult heart rates by multiplying each number by 10. For example, an RPE score of 10 implies a heart rate of around 100 bpm. The basic assumption in the scale is an accuracy of ±10 bpm. Therefore, when someone is exercising at a particular intensity and describes it as 11 on the Borg scale (fairly light), the heart rate should be between 100 and 120 bpm. In recognition of the fact that some people cannot get their hearts to beat at 190 to 200 bpm, the scale has undergone some revision and is now often described as a 10-point scale. Using similar verbal cues, we can also get a sense of work rate using perceived effort. The RPE scale has increased usefulness for people whose heart rates vary significantly from the norm.

Coach Benson has done a lot of work in the area of perceived effort and developed a series of effort-based training tables specifically for runners. Table 2.1 is his adaptation of Borg's Scale for runners. Use it to verify your results if you use the running field test described in chapter 10 to determine your MHR.

Whether you use the Benson table or the Borg chart, combining the common sense of feeling the exertion and effort with your heart rates will allow you both intuitively and objectively to select the right intensity to meet your exercise goal. Eventually, you'll be able to say fairly accurately what your heart rate is, based solely on how you feel. One final point about using this combination method: On days when the conditions of your workout are not normal (e.g., you're still not recovered or it's really humid and warm), the perception approach can be used to reinforce the accuracy of the higher-than-normal heart rates on your heart rate monitor, allowing you to make sensible adjustments to your workout volume and intensity.

TABLE 2.1 Perceived Effort Chart for Runners			
Rating	**Percent effort**	**Perceived exertion**	**Notes**
6	20% effort		Phase I (endurance)
7	30% effort	Very, very light	
8	40% effort		
9	50% effort	Very light	Gentle walk
10	55% effort		
11	60% effort	Fairly light	
12	65% effort		
13	70% effort	Somewhat hard	Steady pace
14	75% effort		Phase II (stamina)
15	80% effort	Hard	
16	85% effort		Phase III (economy)
17	90% effort	Very hard	
18	95% effort		Phase IV (speed)
19	100% effort	Very, very hard	
20	Exhaustion		

Factors Affecting Heart Rate at Rest and During Exercise

One of the most valuable long-term pieces of information you can gather is resting heart rate. When you wake up each morning, take a minute to get an accurate resting heart rate and keep a log. You'll find this an invaluable tool, providing feedback on injury, illness, overtraining, stress, incomplete recovery, and so on. It is also a very simple gauge of improvements in fitness. We know athletes who have gathered resting heart rate data for years and in a day or two can identify a 1 or 2 bpm elevation that precedes an illness or a bonk session. Some newer heart rate monitors have the capacity for 24-hour monitoring, which we'll discuss more in chapter 3.

Several factors affect heart rate at rest and during exercise. In general, the main factors affecting heart rate at rest are fitness and state of recovery. Gender also is suggested to play a role, albeit inconsistently (more about this later). In general, fitter people tend to have lower resting heart rates. Some great athletes of the past have recorded remarkably low resting heart rates. For example, Miguel Indurain, five-time winner of the Tour de France, reported a resting heart rate of only 28 bpm. The reason for this is that, with appropriate training, the heart muscle increases in both size and strength.

The stronger heart moves more blood with each beat (this is called stroke volume) and therefore can do the same amount of work with fewer beats. As you get fitter, your resting heart rate should get lower.

The second main factor affecting resting heart rate is state of recovery. After exercise, particularly after a long run or bike ride, several things happen in the body. Fuel sources are depleted, temperature increases, and muscles are damaged. All of these factors must be addressed and corrected. The body has to work harder, and this increased work results in a higher heart rate. Even though you might feel okay at rest, your body is working harder to repair itself, and you'll notice an elevated heart rate. Monitoring your resting heart rate and your exercise heart rate will allow you to make appropriate adjustments such as eating more or taking a day off when your rate is elevated.

These same factors of recovery and injury also affect heart rate during exercise. The factors that elevate resting heart rate also elevate exercise heart rate. If you're not fully recovered from a previous workout, you might notice, for example, at your usual steady-state pace, an exercise heart rate that is 5 to 10 bpm higher than normal. This is usually accompanied by a rapidly increasing heart rate throughout the exercise session.

An extremely important factor affecting exercise heart rate is temperature. Warmer temperatures cause the heart to beat faster and place considerable strain on the body. Simply put, when it is hot, the body must move more blood to the skin to cool it while also maintaining blood flow to the muscles. The only way to do both of these things is to increase overall blood flow, which means that the heart must beat faster. Depending on how fit you are and how hot it is, this might mean a heart rate that is 20 to 40 bpm higher than normal. Fluid intake is very important under these conditions. Sweating changes blood volume, which eventually can cause cardiac problems. The simplest and most effective intervention to address high temperature and heart rate is regular fluid intake. This helps to preserve the blood volume and prevent the heart from beating faster and faster.

Another important factor affecting exercise heart rate is age. In general, MHR will decline by about 1 beat per year starting at around 20 years old. Interestingly, resting heart rate is not affected. This is why the basic prediction equation of 220 − age has an age correction factor. As a side note, this decrease in MHR often is used to explain decreases in $\dot{V}O_2max$ and endurance performance with increasing age, because the number of times the heart beats in a minute affects how much blood is moved and available to the muscles. We have coached and tested thousands of athletes, and the general trend is that athletes of the same age who produce higher heart rates often have higher fitness scores. However, your MHR is what it is, and you cannot change it. Don't obsess over it.

A final factor is gender. Recent studies have suggested a variation in MHR between males and females. However, the data are inconclusive with the calculations resulting in lower MHRs for males versus females of the same age, while anecdotal reports suggest that the MHRs are actually higher in males. In general, females have smaller hearts and smaller muscles overall than males. Both of these factors would support the conclusion of a higher MHR in females, certainly at the same workload. We have to conclude that the jury is still out on the gender effect.

Chapter 3 considers possible sources of mechanical interference that cause irregular and incorrect readings. However, during exercise, several conditions can develop, often as a result of environmental factors that have a paradoxical but real effect on heart rate. Let's look more specifically at some of these.

Atrial Fibrillation

One medical condition that may cause heart rate irregularity is atrial fibrillation. Although it happens rarely, electrolytes (minerals in the blood that are responsible for the contraction and relaxation of muscles) can be out of balance enough to cause atrial fibrillation, an arrhythmia of the receiving chambers of the heart. This is not immediately life threatening. But, because A-fib is a serious condition, if your numbers are erratic, you should be tested by a cardiologist to determine whether you have this condition.

Typically, people with A-fib have numbers skipping wildly and ranging as much as 30 to 70 bpm higher than expected at a given intensity. They also feel a little faint, weak, and short of breath. If your receiver has the little silhouette of a heart that flashes on and off, study it for a minute or so. If you notice pauses and then several quick flashes of the heart in a row, you should see a physician for a checkup. We've seen several cases of dehydrated runners with A-fib cured quickly by Gatorade, Dr. Cade's wonderful over-the-counter prescription for fluid and electrolyte imbalance.

Atrial fibrillation is one of the more extreme and concerning situations; most sources of interference can be easily traced to one of the other factors addressed in the following sections.

Cardiac Creep

The technical term for this condition is *cardiovascular drift*. In warm, hot, and humid weather, heart rate can easily climb above upper target limits without any increase in effort. Recent studies have shown that this is not just a simple increase in bpm due to the heart having to work harder as it pushes more blood to the skin to cool the body through sweating. This subtle, gradual increase actually also reflects the decrease in blood volume as water is lost through sweat.

It seems logical that this higher heart rate reflects an increase in the pace of the workout and a rise in the effort. But it is not the only explanation. Your heart is just one component of your cardiovascular system. Beats per minute also are influenced by other factors.

Cardiac creep (see figure 2.1) is a good example of the effect of blood volume on the bpm of the heart. When blood volume is normal, resting and exercise heart rates also will be normal. But when blood volume is low as a

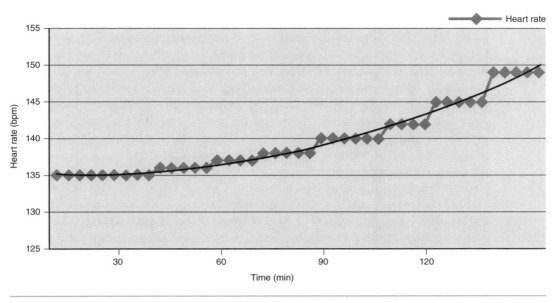

FIGURE 2.1   **Changes in heart rate response over time to a fixed workload.**

result of loss of the water component of blood plasma through sweating, the heart compensates by increasing the frequency of beats to keep the cardiac output constant. This is necessary because cardiac output is determined by the volume of blood ejected with each beat multiplied by the number of times the heart beats per minute. Exercising in warm and humid conditions obviously will make you sweat more than exercising in the cold. We know that you can't rehydrate from water or sport fluids as fast as you can become dehydrated. (Adults can digest and absorb only 6 to 8 ounces of water every 15 to 20 minutes [about 24 ounces in an hour] whereas a well-trained, vigorously exercising person can lose as much as 40 to 50 ounces of water per hour.) To make up for the diminishing amount of blood returning to the heart, the rate is simply increased. Now we don't want to state the obvious, but in warm conditions adequate fluid replacement helps to preserve blood volume and also keep heart rate lower.

Our main point is this: The increase in heart rate can be independent of the effort skeletal muscles are making. A slow, steady increase in heart rate while you are keeping the effort absolutely constant doesn't necessarily mean that you are working harder and that you should therefore ease up or slow down. What you are actually trying to measure by checking your heart rate is how much oxygen the working muscles require. What you really want to know is how hard your body is working, not just how fast your heart is beating. In warm and humid conditions, during longer but easy to barely moderate efforts, a creeping heart rate probably is creating false feedback. If the effort honestly feels the same, but your heart rate has drifted up over your easy-day target by as much as 10 to 15 bpm, you are experiencing cardiac creep.

Easy exercise done in warm, humid conditions might see a heart rate creep as high as 10 to 20 beats above the target zone without actually reflecting an increase in the work rate. On the other hand, hard workouts in warm, humid weather that are planned to take you to or above your anaerobic threshold are not going to be as fast as planned. Once this increase in heart rate cannot keep up with the rapidly diminishing blood volume, your performance will decrease. Your availability of oxygen decreases, causing the muscles to start producing more lactic acid. Now your muscles tighten up and refuse to relax and stretch easily through the range of motion you were enjoying. Slowing down is inevitable as you try to get closer to an aerobically sustainable pace. Now you know why world records aren't set on hot days.

This situation is likely to happen only a few times when you are initially exposed to warmer temperatures. We often see it happen in runs and races early in the month of May when we haven't seen warm temperatures for a while. After two or three weeks of exposure to the warmer temperatures, we tend to see less cardiac creep.

Cardiac Crimp

The converse of cardiac creep is cardiac crimp. On cool days with low humidity when you are supposed to be taking it slow and easy, you can be fooled into allowing low numbers to give you permission to go much faster, and hence much harder, than you should. Don't fall for this. Use your sense of perceived exertion to keep your pace slow and easy. In fact, if the purpose of the workout is recovery, your bpm can never be too low. Celebrate easy effort and low numbers as you think about what happens on hard days. Cool, dry weather results in low heart rates because you are not losing blood volume and you are also cooling very effectively as a result of the low humidity. Think about those workouts on early spring or fall mornings. These conditions are actually perfect for great personal records. You could say: No sweat equals world records and personal records.

Lead Legs

You go out for a run without realizing that you are not recovered, or worse, are starting to become overtrained. You start moving along and quickly perceive the effort to be pretty hard. You check your receiver for validation, expecting to see a high number, but your heart rate is surprisingly low. Next you check your pace, but it's also surprisingly slow.

In this scenario, the fact is that your muscles simply don't have enough energy to move you as fast as you expect. Slow pace equals low heart rate despite your perception of hard effort. So take the day off. Return home and get back in bed. Eat more wisely and drink more profusely. This is not the time to be stubbornly heroic and continue to push through the rest of the workout.

The exercise heart rate response in this mildly overtrained or unrecovered state is best used in conjunction with a waking morning heart rate. If you are indeed not recovered, you should notice two things: an elevated heart rate upon waking and a decreased heart rate during exercise. Remember, with heart rate training it's your body, not your mind, that you want to train. The mental toughening needs to be done on days when you are well rested and can go fast until you drop from exhaustion. Fast times in practice on hard days build confidence as well as improve fitness. If you are a veteran, keep in mind that the best places for fast, hard efforts are races. If you are a rookie, all-out workouts are probably necessary to help you learn what drop-dead exhaustion feels like.

Emotional and Hormonal Changes

We have all felt that racing heart rate in anticipation of a race or competition. In this situation the increase in heart rate is mediated by hormonal responses, primarily adrenaline released as a result of nervousness or excitement. Such elevations in heart rate are confusing and can be difficult to deal with in these situations. You must be alert to this effect and implement strategies such as following a certain warm-up or using breathing exercises or relaxation to control your heart rate response. If adrenaline is increasing your heart rate, your heart rate is not reliable for guiding your effort. This tends to improve with practice.

Recommendations for Evaluating and Revising Zones

By now you know what you need to perform calculations and determine your training zones. You know the factors that will influence your numbers either artificially or because of anatomical or biochemical adaptations. Artificial factors generally go away on their own, but you need to pay attention to the anatomical and biochemical ones because they require that you recalculate some numbers.

Remember that the purpose of training is to induce adaptations in your cardiovascular and respiratory systems and musculature. Some of the changes you want to see are a decrease in your resting heart rate, a decrease in your exercise heart rate at a fixed load, and an increase in your heart rate at anaerobic threshold. The change in resting heart rate is easily explained: the heart is bigger and stronger and can pump more blood with each beat allowing it to beat slower. This factor also explains why the heart rate is lower at a given workload after training. These changes don't necessarily require any recalculations because, to produce heart rates in a given zone, you'll have to move faster and faster, which is exactly what we want.

The number that will need continual monitoring is the heart rate at anaerobic threshold. If all goes according to plan, this heart rate number will increase (e.g., from 145 to 155 bpm) allowing you to move at a faster speed while not putting yourself under any additional metabolic stress such as increased lactic acid. You are now a faster, more efficient machine. This self-correction is the beauty of heart rate training. As we mentioned before, keeping a daily log that tracks both resting and exercise heart rates (along with speed) will allow you to see your progress in several areas. You'll see your heart rate response to a given workload or speed decrease over time, you'll see your speed at a given heart rate increase over time, and finally, you'll see a decrease in your resting heart rate. Self-testing every 10 to 12 weeks will allow you to confirm this information and hopefully notice changes.

After 12 to 16 weeks of training, you should notice the following:

- You are moving at a much faster speed but at the same comfort level.
- You are eliciting a higher heart rate but with the same comfort level.
- Your performance has improved.
- You have to adjust your pace per mile for your aerobic or anaerobic workouts.

In general, we recommend that you revisit your heart rate data every six weeks, especially any time you increase mileage or intensity. This goes back to good record keeping. Keeping an accurate morning and exercise log will be a great help as you plan and monitor your fitness programs.

Getting the Most From Your Monitor

Incorrect heart rate information can come from two sources. The first is incorrect training zone numbers. This might be the case if your predicted maximum heart rate (MHR) is different from your actual MHR. Also, the monitor itself may be displaying erroneous numbers because of poor contact or another technical problem. Awareness of the origin of the error usually leads to an easy fix. This book mostly addresses using your heart rate to optimize training; however, you need to be sure that the data you get from your monitor are accurate.

Watching Your Numbers

As you learned in chapter 1, using heart rate to guide your training is a sound, scientific way to ensure that you train at the right intensity at the right time. It is also time efficient, helping you avoid garbage work you don't need so you can meet the objective of your workout. Much of this chapter is devoted to making sure that you aren't wasting time blindly staying in heart rate zones that aren't effective or valid.

Before relying on your heart rate monitor, take it out for a trial workout to get a rough idea of how it works and the sort of feedback it gives you. Before using it for another workout, closely study the information in this chapter and chapter 2 to guarantee that you are using your monitor correctly.

The first thing you want to do is ensure that the monitor is fitted correctly. Strap it on and make sure it contacts your skin properly by holding the rubber transmitter section with the electrodes on your chest just below your chest muscles. With your free hand, bring the elastic strap from behind your back and around your other side, without stretching the elastic material, to within 6 inches (15 cm) of the free end of the transmitter section. If the elastic strap is too far away or too close, adjust it through the slide until you have that crucial 6-inch (15 cm) gap between the end of the chest unit. Now pull and stretch the elastic strap until you can clip the end into the transmitter section. It should feel snug, but not so tight that it restricts the expansion of your rib cage as you inhale. If the strap is too loose, the transmitter unit will slip up and down on your skin and create friction that will result in phony numbers being sent to your wrist receiver. You may have to moisten the grooved electrodes to start the conduction of the electrical activity of your beating heart to the transmitter.

Now, go for nice 20- to 30-minute very comfortable walk or jog at a conversational pace. Observe the heart rate numbers and mentally note them along with how you feel. If your monitor has a split time recording function, press the button at random times while walking or jogging.

When you finish, hit the recall functions and get the high and low numbers and the average heart rate for the session. Write them down, along with a verbal description of the effort you felt at those recorded points (e.g., light, very light, somewhat hard).

The heart rate monitor is a machine, and like all machines, it is a bit temperamental. To use it properly, you need to be aware of the factors that affect

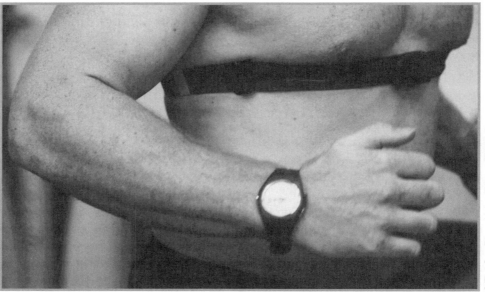

© The San Diego Union-Tribune/ZUMA Press

To get the most from your heart rate monitor, attach it correctly, use it frequently, and understand its strengths and limitations.

the monitor, the heart rate response, and ultimately the information from the monitor. Chapter 2 covered some specific issues that affect heart rate zones and readings. You should not proceed if you have not resolved these issues to your satisfaction. However, other conditions can cause your monitor to display results that appear to be anomalies, contradictions, and paradoxes. Before you send it to the repair shop, closely review the information in this chapter. Almost all the brands and models of heart rate monitors we have used are very reliable and accurate. Therefore, when your numbers seem to make no sense at all, your best action would be to check out the conditions and situations discussed in this chapter. You are most likely getting false readings, so don't worry.

As you learned in chapter 1, individualizing your target heart rate zones to fit the objectives of your workouts is as important and challenging as individualizing your workouts to suit yourself. Once you know for sure what your MHR is, and once you have carefully calculated your target heart rate zones for each of the workouts you want to do, then read on. If you strap on your monitor and go without knowing what the numbers should be telling you, you'll get frustrated. Please don't give up on this investment. It may take longer than you expected to get started, but without doing this work now, our answer to your question "What about me?" will not make sense.

Here are some warnings about contradictory and paradoxical numbers that could cause you to sprint when you should jog, put the brakes on when you should pedal harder, or think that your irregular pulse must surely be a heart attack. By understanding the physical or mechanical causes of these numbers, you'll know that you can just relax while using the common sense of perceived exertion to figure out whether what you're seeing is valid.

Reluctant Readings

If you strap on the transmitter and do not see a reading on the receiver, the electrodes are probably not in solid contact with your skin. Wet your finger with water or saliva and moisten the electrodes. Or just start working out and, as soon as you sweat, the readings will pop up.

Technical Difficulties That Cause Irregular Numbers

Several conditions may cause your heart rate numbers to skip all over the place. Normally, you will notice a steady increase or decrease in your heart rate that will pretty much match your effort. The heart rate monitor is not an electrocardiogram (ECG). However, it does use the electrical activity of the heart to give you a signal. Therefore, any time an irregularity occurs in the signal, it will be reflected in the heart rate number displayed.

Slippage

One cause of irregular readings is a loose chest strap that allows the electrodes to slip and slide on the skin and cause electricity from the friction. This interferes with the transmitting of the electrical impulses of the heart muscle. You need to shorten the elastic strap. If you have a very small rib cage and narrow chest, just tighten the strap well past the halfway point to achieve the 6-inch (15 cm) gap even if it means that the extra material loops down. Put a safety pin in front of the slide to keep the strap from slipping back to the original halfway position. If this is a consistent problem, buy a shorter strap or permanently shorten your strap by putting a few stitches into it to hold it in the shortened position. Straps stretch over time and become loose. When this happens, we recommend buying a new strap.

Static Cling on Clothing

One cause of irregular readings is clothing worn over the transmitter. Shirts still charged with static electricity from the dryer can confuse the receiver. Nylon wind jackets can generate static electricity that also can interfere with the transmission from the chest strap to the receiver, although this is more likely to be a concern in dry or cold climates. Usually, sweat takes care of it pretty quickly. Females may find that underwire bras can be a source of interference. If you suspect that static cling is causing the problem, wet your hand and wipe it across the material in front of the transmitter, or just wait until you've run far enough for sweat to drain off the static. (This should take 8 to 10 minutes.) The signal is also transmitted better and stronger once you start to sweat.

Interference From Cross Feeds

Cross feed occurs when your monitor receives information from the transmitter of the person next to you. The solution may be to find a partner who isn't as scientific as you are (and therefore does not wear a monitor). If not, arrange yourselves so that you are both wearing your receivers on your outside arms. More advanced (and expensive) monitors have their own embedded codes to prevent cross feeds.

If you're a real techno geek, you may have other devices that are confusing your heart rate signal. When testing in the lab, we have seen devices such as pedometers and GPS systems interfere with the heart rate monitor signal. This is also the case when exercising indoors on a stationary piece of equipment with lots of information displayed on the console. In this case, either exercise outside for a change or take the receiver off your wrist and strap it to a lower part of the machine out of range of the console.

Soaked Shirts

Shirts soaked with sweat can get heavy enough to bounce up and down in front of your transmitter and interfere with the signal to your receiver. If it is that hot and humid, remove the chest strap from under your shirt and refasten it on top of the wet shirt just below your chest muscles. The wet shirt will still allow the electrodes to have great contact with skin and be able to pick up the electrical activity of your heart muscles. In fact, this is also the solution if you experience chaffing from a strap that seems to slip up and down on your skin. Just wet your shirt first before starting the workout.

Safety Alarms

Radio frequency alarm systems installed in buildings can occasionally interfere with your monitor's own radio frequency as you go past. The solution: ignore them and keep going. The goofy numbers will return to normal as soon as you are out of range of the alarm system.

New Technology

Heart rate monitors have advanced dramatically in the last five years. They have improved in function, appearance, reliability, and accuracy. Modern monitors provide information on calorie expenditure, oxygen consumption, time in target zones, maximum heart rate achieved during the workout, and heart rate recovery zones, as well as audible signals, 24-hour heart rate measurements, and a whole lot more.

Calories expended, which is indirectly calculated from heart rate, is a helpful feature because it expands the usage of the monitor to populations that are less performance oriented and more interested in issues such as health improvement, weight loss, and cardiac rehabilitation.

For athletes, the 24-hour monitoring option provides an abundance of new information that they can use to fine-tune their programs and monitor their intensity levels. This fairly noninvasive system tracks not only exercise heart rates but also recovery rates. This provides vital information related to adaptation and recovery. By tracking the heart rate over 24 hours, athletes gets thousands of data points that are downloadable to a computer to create a graph or spreadsheet. These data can reveal the slightest signs of illness, overtraining, fatigue, and improvement. Prior to this option, athletes were unable to detect the small, subtle differences that revealed these problems until they caused disruption or system failure.

Of course, with increased function comes increased complexity and cost. However, spending a little time with the owner's manual will resolve most operating concerns, and ensuring that the watch is properly set up and programmed from the outset will result in much greater accuracy. Many features are downloadable with more advanced systems. Being able to download and observe the heart rate responses to a single exercise session is valuable. You can look back at particular times of a workout or a hill or a longer workout and detect where your creep really set in, a very entertaining way to distract yourself during longer workouts.

Deciding which heart rate monitor to buy is really a matter of personal choice. Factors that will influence your decision include cost, your goals, your fitness level, and the amount of information you really need. The more serious and competitive you are, the more features you'll want. Features such as 24-hour monitoring, caloric expenditure, and target zone audible alarm signals can increase the accuracy and individualization of your training program. Many heart rate monitor company Web sites provide sheets that compare their models to their competitors' to allow you to see at a glance the different features of the models.

A final consideration when purchasing your heart rate monitor is that some companies make models with additional features that span different sports. For example, if you are a triathlete, you may want a heart rate monitor with a built-in GPS system that allows you to record speeds and distances travelled. These are very helpful features.

Now you know all the bits and pieces that can affect the way heart rate monitors work, and you have a much greater understanding of their capabilities and can appreciate the information at your fingertips. Understanding all these features will allow you to plan better workouts and then adjust your intensities. The information you get will be based on you and will allow you to plan and evaluate using multiple criteria. In the next chapters, we start to look at how to use the heart rate monitor when putting the theory into practice.

PART II

TRAINING

CHAPTER 4

Targeting Sport-Specific Fitness With Heart Rate

From your own experiences with exercise, you know that there are different types of fitness. Some people are better at biking than swimming, some people are better at speed than distance, some people are very strong but can't run very far. Basically, these different situations require different types of fitness, which we discuss later in the chapter in terms of different energy systems. The more common terms you may be familiar with are *aerobic* and *anaerobic*, which in simple terms refer to longer, slower exercise (aerobic) and shorter, faster exercise (anaerobic).

The way people move in different sports reveals that different sports have different fitness requirements and therefore different energy needs. For example, the soccer player is constantly starting and stopping or jogging and sprinting, the tennis player is stopping and starting rapidly, and the distance runner exercises at the same speed continuously. Because sports require different movement patterns, they require different types of training. To understand the various phases of your training program, you must have a basic understanding of the different types of fitness and the energy systems they use. If you are an endurance athlete, you also need to understand the factors that affect the way these energy systems operate. Two main factors are nutrition and intensity. Even though our main focus in this book is heart rate training, in this chapter we take a more detailed look at how other peripheral factors influence your ability.

Understanding Energy Production

Heart rate response to exercise is governed by numerous factors, the cardiovascular, or circulatory, system being one. Therefore, our focus on heart rate must also include work done by the complete cardiovascular system. This system delivers both oxygen and energy to the muscles. We refer to this use of energy as the metabolic capacity of the muscles.

The two basic metabolic energy systems are the aerobic system and the anaerobic system. Each primarily uses different fuels for energy, and your success at getting into shape or competing depends on how well trained a particular energy system is. In general, longer, slower activities such as cross-country skiing and distance running depend heavily on the aerobic system and primarily convert fat into energy. Sprint and explosive events, such as the 100 meters or hammer throw, rely heavily on the anaerobic system. Team sports fall in between because they use both, although team sports are quite varied in their reliance on these energy systems. For example, ice hockey is 80 to 90 percent anaerobic and 10 to 20 percent aerobic, whereas soccer is around 50/50. Table 4.1 shows the use of aerobic and anaerobic energy in several sports.

These metabolic requirements have implications for the way you train. Too much or too little emphasis on a particular energy system will compromise not only your performance but also your recovery and risk of injury.

TABLE 4.1 Aerobic and Anaerobic Energy Usage in Several Sports

Sport	Aerobic %	Anaerobic %
Soccer	50%	50%
Ice hockey	10–20	80–90
Rowing	70	30
Marathon	90	10
Cross-country skiing	97.5	2.5
100 m running	5	95
Distance swimming	70	30
Road cycling	80	20

Three Energy Systems

The ultimate source of energy in muscles is adenosine triphosphate, or ATP. No matter what you eat or drink, it must ultimately be converted to ATP before it can be used as energy. The body delivers ATP through three energy systems: the ATP-PC system, the anaerobic glycolysis system, and the aerobic system. (Note that the first two are anaerobic systems.) Typically, one energy system predominates at any given intensity, but all three contribute at least some energy during any exercise.

Monitoring heart rate is significantly easier and more reliable during aerobic exercise than it is during exercise that relies on either of the two anaerobic systems. That is not to say that we cannot use it to monitor anaerobic work, because we can—at the lower end of anaerobic exercise it can be quite reliable. However, as intensities increase and we get to the high end of anaerobic exercise, there is a delay in the heart rate response, especially if intensity increases rapidly. This delay detracts from its reliability. However, when this delay happens, the reliability of the recovery heart rate to gauge when to ramp back up again actually increases. This is an added benefit of heart rate training. Therefore, in these situations, the heart rate monitor is perhaps best used as a recovery tool.

ATP-PC System   The ATP-PC system is a very powerful, high-energy system capable of delivering huge amounts of energy rapidly. However, it can last only for a few seconds. It is recruited mainly for sprinting and other high-speed changes. It requires maximum or near maximum efforts for the most part. However, it is also the predominant energy system used during the first few seconds of any exercise regardless of intensity. This energy system relies on ATP that is stored in the muscle, which is then released rapidly when needed. The system is highly dependent on creatine phosphate, which is why power and speed athletes often supplement with creatine. The system can recover quickly, usually within three to five minutes.

Exercise heart rate is of little use when exercising predominantly within the ATP-PC system because the work is over very rapidly and the heart rate response lags way behind the work effort. As with work within the anaerobic glycolysis system, heart rate monitoring is better used here for gauging recovery here.

Anaerobic Glycolysis System   The anaerobic glycolysis system also may be referred to as the glycolytic system or lactic acid system. Modern exercise science now refers to it as either fast or slow glycolysis. This system is recruited predominantly during maximum exercise that lasts 15 to 90 seconds. The system relies on the breakdown of carbohydrates and can provide energy fairly rapidly. However, this reliance on carbohydrates often results in the production of lactic acid, which is why the system sometimes is called the lactic acid system. When oxygen levels are insufficient to facilitate a complete breakdown of carbohydrates (or the energy is being produced quickly), lactic acid is the end product. As the lactic acid accumulates, it creates an acidic environment that causes the legs to get heavy and muscle contraction to be impaired. Often, you get this sensation after running or cycling up a hill. You are probably familiar with that feeling of heavy legs. As the intensity decreases after this initial effort, your muscle can then buffer the lactic acid and allow you to go on your way.

Relating heart rate to training in these shorter anaerobic sessions is a little more difficult because the time it takes the heart rate to respond and reflect the work rate can sometimes be as long as the exercise bout itself. Therefore, in the shorter sessions (less than 90 seconds) we advise that you use heart rate to gauge your recovery interval more than your actual work rate. As the work increases in length, beyond 90 seconds but still fairly anaerobic, your heart rate will provide better feedback.

Aerobic System The final energy system is the aerobic system, or oxidative system, which pretty much has an unlimited supply of energy. It burns mainly fat. The average adult has about 100,000 calories of fat, although some of us have a little more. The aerobic system produces energy slowly but has great capacity and can go for hours and hours. Because exercise is performed at a more moderate intensity, plenty of oxygen is available, and fat, which takes longer to break down, can be metabolized. That is why endurance athletes often are thinner, leaner, and lighter.

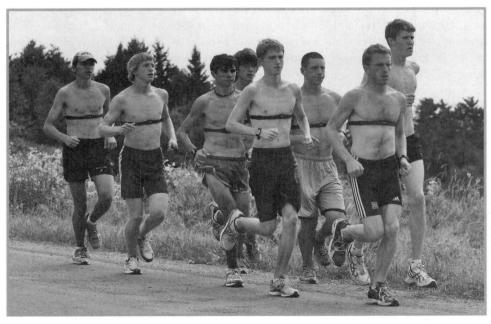

Photo courtesy of Michael Cohen

Aerobic exercise performed at an intensity below 75 percent MHR burns fat, which explains why endurance athletes, such as runners, tend to be leaner.

In terms of heart rate training zones, the aerobic system predominates at intensities below 75 percent of maximum heart rate (MHR).

Our challenge is to put energy systems into the context of heart rate training zones. How hard or at what intensity as a percentage of MHR do you need to exercise to challenge a particular energy system? What fuels are you burning and in what ratios at any given intensity? What duration parameters are associated with these energy systems? To answer these questions, we need to look at these systems in a little more detail.

Energy Systems During Exercise

It is useful to think about the energy systems in terms of time parameters. If you exercise maximally for 15 seconds, then 90 seconds, and then 5 minutes, you would have a nice spectrum of the energy systems (see table 4.2). All-out exercise that lasts less than 15 seconds predominantly uses the ATP-PC system. All-out exercise lasting 15 to 90 seconds predominantly uses anaerobic glycolysis. And all-out exercise lasting more than 90 seconds predominantly uses the aerobic system. Track and field events illustrate this continuum. Table 4.3 shows track events along with their predominant energy systems.

Athletes are leaner as the distances get longer, indicating more fat-burning aerobic work. Athletes who are better at shorter distances are more muscular and well defined. We will talk more about this later. Table 4.1 (page 46) shows a metabolic breakdown of some other sports.

TABLE 4.2 Energy Systems by Duration of Exercise

Energy system	Duration (in seconds)
ATP-PC	1–15
Anaerobic glycolysis	15–90
Aerobic	>90

TABLE 4.3 Energy Systems Used in Track Events

Track event	Energy system	World record
100 m	ATP-PC	9.58 seconds
200 m	ATP-PC	19.19 seconds
400 m	Anaerobic glycolysis	43.18 seconds
800 m	Anaerobic glycolysis	1:41:01 minutes
1,500 m	Aerobic	3:26:00 minutes
3,000 m	Aerobic	7:20:67 minutes

Nutritional Considerations in Energy Supply

The energy system used is tightly linked to a particular nutrient such as carbohydrate, fat, or protein. Simply put, the aerobic system relies on fat, whereas the aerobic glycolysis system relies on carbohydrate and protein. The ATP-PC system relies on ATP stored in the muscle and must have the stores replenished immediately after a maximal bout. This replenishment occurs via aerobic metabolism.

Regardless of the type of exercise you do, recovery is always aerobic even though it may require carbohydrate replenishment, as is the case after long runs or bike rides. The anaerobic glycolysis system relies primarily on carbohydrate and a small amount of protein. However, this system is also active during aerobic exercise. Running out of carbohydrate during an aerobic event (also known as hitting the wall, bonking, or crashing) is a function of low carbohydrate levels. Although many people think aerobic exercise is just fat burning, it also uses a lot of carbohydrate. This is why long endurance events require adequate carbohydrate replacement.

Fitness Needs of Different Sports

An understanding of energy systems clarifies why athletes in different sports have to train in different ways. A linebacker in American football trains very differently from a 2,000-meter rower because training programs must stimulate and simulate the energy systems that predominate during competitions. This explains why certain body types are common in certain sports. Lean, light athletes usually have better-trained aerobic systems; bigger, more muscular athletes usually are better trained anaerobically. So soccer players have different physiques from rugby players, sprinters, and endurance athletes.

A final consideration is the relationship of muscle fiber types to energy metabolism. Slow-twitch fibers, which are of benefit in endurance activities, prefer to burn fat. They also are smaller and leaner. Fast-twitch muscle fibers, which are of benefit during power and speed activities, prefer to burn carbohydrate. Fast-twitch fibers also are bigger and thicker.

Heart Rate Monitoring Across Energy Systems

Now that you understand the three energy systems and the intensity associated with each one, you can design your workouts to stimulate energy systems by selecting appropriate heart rates. This definitely works best for determining intensities for the anaerobic glycolysis system and the aerobic system, but has limited use during maximum, short-term, high-intensity exercise such as sprinting. However, heart rate is extremely useful in gauging recovery profiles during short-term, high-intensity bouts (which use both the ATP-PC and the anaerobic glycolysis systems) because you can determine

Understanding Muscle Fiber Types

Muscle fiber type is a frequent topic of discussion among athletes. In particular, athletes are interested in whether they can change fiber type to ultimately improve performance. The human body is composed of two basic fiber types: fast-twitch and slow-twitch. Slow-twitch fibers are often referred to as type I fibers. Fast-twitch fibers often are divided into two subcategories: type IIa and type IIb.

Fibers are classified this way because of the nature of the activity that recruits them. Fast-twitch fibers are recruited during fast, explosive movements. Slow-twitch fibers are recruited for less intense contractions. The fibers themselves are inherently different, and understanding this difference is vital in designing an appropriate training program. Perhaps the two most important factors to understand about muscle fibers are their biochemical differences and the intensity of muscle contraction and fiber recruitment.

Biochemical characteristics are important because they determine how the muscle must be exercised to induce adaptation. The two types of fibers are metabolically different. When you exercise aerobically, you are mainly using slow-twitch fibers (type I). When you exercise anaerobically, you are mainly using fast-twitch fibers (types IIa and IIb). Slow-twitch fibers (type I) are more fatigue resistant than fast-twitch fibers (types IIa and IIb). Therefore, specificity in training is crucial for causing biochemical adaptation within fiber groups.

The differences in fiber makeup also explain why particular fibers can work longer or harder, which is determined by the duration and intensity of exercise. Therefore, targeting fiber types during training by selecting the right intensity or duration is a must to ensure progress.

One other consideration is that fast-twitch fibers prefer to burn carbohydrate. Burning carbohydrate tends to produce the infamous lactate, which, if allowed to accumulate, ultimately will slow you down. In contrast, slow-twitch fibers prefer to burn fat and require lots of oxygen. That is why at lower intensities more energy comes from fat stores. As the time of exercise increases to three, four, or five hours or more, you must slow down to ensure that you have enough energy reserves to last.

On average, adults store about 2,000 calories of carbohydrate and 80,000 to 100,000 calories of fat. Exercising at a moderate to hard intensity burns about 750 calories per hour, most of it carbohydrate. That's why people often bonk two or three hours into a session. Believe it or not, your basic fitness goal is to improve your efficiency at burning fat. In the field, we use the term *glycogen sparing*. However, don't be fooled into developing only your aerobic capacity. You need good anaerobic and aerobic capacity to be a good endurance athlete.

To induce fast-twitch fiber adaptation, or anaerobic capacity, you must exercise at high intensities. The opposite holds true for slow-twitch adaptation, or aerobic capacity. But what is high intensity? A lack of understanding of high intensity is where many athletes fall short; they don't exercise at a high enough intensity. An intensity of 90 percent MHR recruits only about 85 percent of the available fast-twitch fibers. Even 100 percent intensity recruits only about 95 percent of the available fast-twitch fibers. As intensity decreases, greater slow-twitch recruitment occurs. At 70 percent intensity, only about 10 percent of the available fast-twitch fibers are recruited. The bottom line: Fast-twitch fiber recruitment is difficult to attain and requires highly intense activity.

(continued)

Understanding Muscle Fiber Types *(continued)*

So do endurance athletes need to develop anaerobic ability? Absolutely. All else being equal, the more powerful athlete is always the better athlete. Top-class aerobic performance in competition often is determined by anaerobic capability. When you put in that final sprint or little burst in the middle of a race, your anaerobic capacity picks up that energy demand. This is why you must train these fibers specifically during practice.

So does your fiber type distribution determine your potential? Basically, yes. International-class athletes in endurance sports demonstrate greater percentages of slow-twitch than of fast-twitch fibers. The opposite is true of power and speed athletes. Top-class sprinters may demonstrate up to 75 percent fast-twitch fibers, whereas top-class endurance athletes, such as cross-country skiers, may demonstrate up to 90 percent slow-twitch. For the most part, this distribution is genetically determined; you cannot convert fibers from slow to fast, or vice versa. However, there are intermediate fibers that can, with training, demonstrate characteristics of the fiber types recruited during training, giving a little more reserve in specific situations. You also can improve the potential of existing fibers with appropriate training. Your best bet is to specifically target fiber types during practice and training and to work hard at developing regimes to ensure fast-twitch recruitment. Unfortunately, regimes to improve fast-twitch recruitment are more difficult and less comfortable than others, but the sacrifice will be worth it come competition time.

when you are ready to repeat a sprint or an interval by when your heart rate has recovered to a certain level.

Some coaches deem an athlete ready for a repeat when the heart rate drops below 65 percent MHR following an interval. Unfortunately this approach is underused as recovery heart rates are a very good indicator of overall aerobic conditioning. As you get fitter, you should notice quicker and quicker recoveries between higher-intensity bouts even within exercise sessions. For example, cyclists often achieve near-maximum heart rates on short climbs but then drop back down to 65 to 75 percent within a few minutes indicating good overall aerobic fitness.

To use this heart rate and training information for your training, you need to consider the following:

1. What is the aerobic versus anaerobic breakdown of your sport?

2. How do you allocate a representative amount of time to aerobic and anaerobic work based on your metabolic breakdown?

3. What heart rate zones should you exercise at to cause adaptation and challenge the desired energy system?

4. Should you consider any nutritional intervention to enhance your energy system performance?

5. What recovery heart rates should you be looking for between intervals or after other shorter periods of high intensity?

The answers to these questions will allow you to select the right training intensities for your exercise program.

Increasing Aerobic Endurance

The coming chapters contain general discussions of principles and concepts of heart rate training so you can apply what you have learned so far. They cover the development of the four components of fitness by discussing their places in each of the four phases of training. After you finish these chapters, turn to the chapter that offers you a sample training plan and pattern of workouts for your choice of activity. However, study chapters 5 through 8 in their entirety before trying to implement any of these suggestions. In other words, don't false start by jumping the gun. You need to see the big picture of all the training zones before developing a training plan.

Chapter 5 covers specific exercise intensity levels for developing, enhancing, and maintaining your crucial aerobic endurance base, which is the building block of fitness and recovery for every sport. To help you fully appreciate the importance of endurance training, we also discuss the physical changes needed to develop this critical component of overall fitness.

Whether you are increasing your base endurance or redeveloping it after a layoff from an injury or postseason recovery period, this first, or base, phase of training is critical. Your target heart rate zones will range from 60 to 75 percent of your maximum heart rate (MHR).

The word *aerobic* means "with oxygen" and is associated with the easy, low-intensity effort that develops and maintains endurance. If a workout is easy and slow enough to allow casual conversation, you can rest assured that plenty of oxygen is present in the circulatory system. To be sure that the effort is aerobic, we like to apply the Faulkner test. Can you comfortably carry on conversations that resemble author William Faulkner's writing (which goes on for pages before coming to a period) without the slightest challenge to your breathing? If so, then it's aerobic and you're in your heart rate zone of 60 to 75 percent.

If you are coming back after a layoff to build a new aerobic endurance base, enough time and all efforts in the zone of 60 to 75 percent MHR will get the job done. Such a wide range is appropriate for several reasons, one of which is that you will be working your way back into shape and your heart rate will elevate easily and quickly. Our generous allowance to the top of the endurance range will help you avoid paces that are so slow that you become discouraged.

If you are already in training but are looking to improve your base endurance, efforts in the zone of 75 to 80 percent at steady-state paces will enhance and increase endurance. The upcoming sections explain the difference between developing endurance at 60 to 75 percent effort, enhancing it at 75 to 80 percent, and then maintaining it at both 65 to 70 percent and 60 to 65 percent MHR. But first, let's look at the main goals and adaptations that take place with endurance training.

Physiological Adaptations to Endurance Training

For most people, the bottom-line goal of endurance training is performing faster. Although this may indeed be the net outcome, many microadaptations take place within the body to allow you to perform faster. People vary by body type and in response to stimulus, and the type of training affects the response, which is why we need a varied complement of training approaches. We have selected a few of the adaptations that occur with endurance-type training for discussion.

The physiological changes that occur in athletes are due largely to the combined effects of cardiovascular, respiratory, metabolic, and muscular adaptations. The first and most obvious change is an increase in $\dot{V}O_2$max. This is most simply explained by the Fick equation:

$$\dot{V}O_2\text{max} = \text{MHR} \times \text{SVmax} \times A\dot{V}O_2\text{difference,}$$

in which HR = heart rate, SV = stroke volume (the amount of blood pumped per heart beat), and $A\dot{V}O_2$difference is the difference in O_2 saturation between arterial and venous blood (arteriovenous oxygen difference), which is an indicator of O_2 extraction.

In locker room language, $\dot{V}O_2$max is the combined ability of your respiratory, circulatory, and muscular systems to take in, distribute, and use oxygen.

Oxygen Changes

In the well-trained endurance athlete, MHR actually decreases slightly with progressing fitness. Stroke volume (SV), on the other hand, increases, and $A\dot{V}O_2$ difference increases. These variables primarily explain the adaptation. As a muscle, the heart moves more blood with each beat as it becomes stronger, resulting in a lower resting heart rate. The capillary density of the muscles increases, facilitating more blood and gas transport. The net outcome is an increase in $\dot{V}O_2$max. Long, slow, aerobic, low-intensity work early in a training program promotes this capillary adaptation rather than the kinds of adaptations that take place during higher-intensity workouts after the endurance base is developed.

Endurance training also increases blood volume by expanding plasma volume and increasing the number of red blood cells. The change in plasma volume is due to an increase in water retention, which actually causes a condition called hemodilution (a decrease in red blood cell percentage). However, the absolute numbers are increased, which facilitates more oxygen transport.

Respiratory adaptations also occur. In particular, an increase in maximum voluntary ventilation (MVV) occurs. This allows for a greater volume of air to be moved both in and out of the lungs, facilitating an increase in both carbon dioxide removal and oxygen uptake. This adaptation is explained by improvements in respiratory muscle endurance and economy.

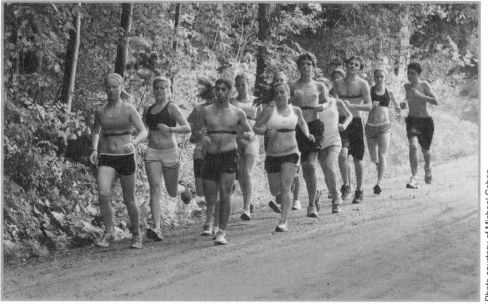

Photo courtesy of Michael Cohen

Endurance training causes many adaptations in the body, including an increase in stroke volume and blood volume, more efficient respiration, and developments in muscle structure that allow the athlete to perform longer before fatiguing.

Muscle Changes

Numerous changes also take place within the muscles as a result of endurance training. There is an increase in both the number and size of mitochondria, the so-called workhorses of the muscle. This adaptation promotes the use of fatty acids, allowing a greater production of energy ATP. This is particularly important for the endurance athlete, because it slows the depletion of body glycogen stores, which are limited. The net result is a longer time to fatigue. The preference for fatty acids over glycogen by the endurance-trained body also results in slower lactic acid accumulation.

You can see how interdependent the body systems are. An increase in respiratory economy and endurance allows for greater carbon dioxide removal and oxygen transport to the blood. An increase in capillary density then facilitates the transport of these gases to the mitochondria in the muscle. The gas diffusion rate at the mitochondria affects not only energy production but also the substrate source for this energy production. As carbohydrate (glycogen) is used more sparingly because of the greater use of fats, time to fatigue is prolonged and lactate accumulation is slowed. The net result is a faster or longer performance.

Several other adaptations also take place as you develop endurance:

- Less carbohydrate is burned and therefore less lactic acid is produced.
- The greater number of blood vessels (those little capillaries) allows for greater removal of metabolic waste products.
- Muscle strength improves.
- Joints, bones, tendons, and ligaments get stronger.
- Efficiency improves.

These and other subtle changes improve a muscle's ability to keep going. Think of it as going long, going slow, and going with someone who talks too much. That's endurance.

The take-home message from this list of myriad adaptations is that a varied training approach is needed to address all the required adaptations. Not only should training be varied, but it should also be sequential because some adaptations are required before others. For example, long, slow work should precede high-intensity work. The following sections explain the progression from developing endurance at 60 to 75 percent MHR, to enhancing endurance at 75 to 80 percent, to maintaining endurance at 65 to 70 percent and 60 to 65 percent.

Endurance Development

To develop and improve endurance in the heart rate zone of 60 to 75 percent MHR, try to spend as much time as close to 75 percent as possible. In the general endurance zone of 60 to 75 percent, the muscle uses a mixture of fat and carbohydrate for fuel. These fuels are supplied at varying ratios depending on the intensity of the activity. For low-intensity endurance activities with lots of oxygen present, the majority of the fuel comes from fat although carbohydrate still provides limited amounts of fuel. However, if the event lasts long enough, the limited supply of carbohydrate stored in the muscle can be depleted. In marathon runners this is known as hitting the wall and happens when the muscle has only fat for its fuel supply. To burn fats cleanly, the body needs lots of oxygen, which forces the runner to slow down. Improving the body's ability to burn fat more efficiently to allow carbohydrate supplies to last until the end of the event is one of the major goals of endurance training. A second one, which we will elaborate on shortly, is the strengthening of the musculoskeletal system.

To demonstrate the importance of oxygen in endurance activities, consider that you draw 95 percent of your fuel from fat and 5 percent from carbohydrate at basal metabolism (when you are in deep sleep and your body is awash with oxygen). However, once you exercise hard enough to elevate your heart rate into the endurance training zone, that ratio quickly changes. For unfit folks, carbohydrate becomes more important as the availability of oxygen decreases. In the 70 to 75 percent heart rate zone, as much as half of the energy comes from carbohydrate. It takes the liver 24 to 48 hours to convert glycogen, the chemical form of carbohydrate stored in the muscles, from various forms of carbohydrate. If you exercise after only 24 hours of recovery (i.e., daily), you will create a short-term glycogen deficit that will then cause muscle enzymes to improve their ability to break down and metabolize fats. This can happen to such a degree that endurance athletes such as long-distance runners and cross-country skiers get as much as 80 percent of their fuel from fat when in the low range of 60 to 70 percent MHR. Have you ever wondered why the great endurance athletes are so thin? One reason is that they burn a lot of fat.

While reaching this stage of energy efficiency, you also will be performing enough aerobic exercise in the 60 to 75 percent zone to cause the adaptations you need in the cardiovascular, respiratory, and muscular systems.

Equally important as the ability of your muscular engine to use fuel is the strength of the transmission, your connective tissues. Ligaments, tendons, bones, cartilage, and joints take much longer than muscles to get stronger because their blood supply is not nearly as rich. Therefore, you need to beware of the dreaded Cadillac engine/Chevy transmission syndrome. Because your powerful muscular engine can easily tear up your delicate connective transmission, you'll be very susceptible to classic overuse injuries such as Achilles' tendonitis, plantar fasciitis, iliotibial band syndrome, and even stress fractures. Avoiding these perils will be covered in later discussions concerning the length of time you need to spend in phase I.

Training Techniques for Developing Endurance

You improve endurance by training in the zone of 60 to 75 percent MHR. The following two training regimens (in order of our preference) will help you achieve this goal:

1. An adaptation of classic fartlek training, which is ideal for initial base building. In this context, let's call it heart rate fartlek so the purists of the Swedish language won't complain. Picture your heart rate roller-coasting up and down.

2. Long, slow distance (commonly known as LSD) for athletes who want to take their base to the next level and increase their aerobic endurance over longer distances or times. Picture someone doing a lot of jogging.

Both of these workouts are practiced within the 60 to 75 percent MHR zone. They can be used singularly or in combination with the base phase of conditioning to develop aerobic endurance. This is what we refer to as getting in shape. Using these approaches will allow you to stimulate your muscles long enough and over long enough periods of time to induce adaptations.

If you are getting in shape or if your level of athletic activity has been interrupted because of personal or medical reasons for several weeks, you

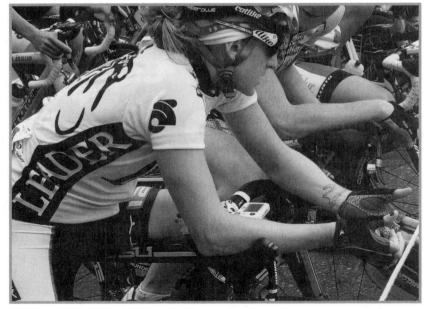

Heart rate fartlek workouts, in which you cycle your heart rate up and down within your training zone, will help you quickly build a base of endurance and prepare for more challenging events, such as races.

will need to redevelop your endurance base. Phase I of conditioning usually takes the average, sedentary adult up to 12 weeks. If you have already been through the conditioning process, you should be able to redevelop an endurance base within six to eight weeks. A shorter period of four weeks should be sufficient to redevelop endurance if you are coming back after a postseason period of active rest. In any case, an adaptation of classic fartlek training is ideal for training in the 60 to 75 percent MHR zone.

If you are rebuilding a new base, take careful note of the following discussion. Our heart rate fartlek workouts are the essence of heart rate monitor training. If you have been fairly active and have had some athletic experience earlier in life, you might consider LSD the most attractive activity for getting back into shape. But please read the following to see how the advantages of monitored training can be applied. Heart rate fartlek training is perfect for whichever activity—jogging, rowing, cycling—you choose. Heart rate fartlek workouts are a great way to introduce small elements of faster movement into your workouts for manageable periods of time and still keep the risk of injury at the absolute minimum.

Our prize-winning adaptation of fartlek training to the heart rate monitor is the perfect example of smart, individualized training. Here's an example of how it would work. For a 20-minute session, you would do the following:

1. Calculate your target heart rate zone with the upper limit at 75 percent and a lower limit at 60 percent MHR.

2. Pick an exercise mode—walking, jogging, running, cycling, rowing, or any of the machines such as the elliptical or stair-climbing types in the aerobic section of your fitness center.

3. Start exercising slowly and easily as your heart rate eases up into your 60 to 75 percent zone. As you warm into the workout, you'll probably find yourself gradually picking up the pace and effort. Your heart rate will rise and eventually hit the 75 percent upper limit.

4. At that point, to keep the workout aerobic, quickly slow down until your heart rate drops back to as close to 60 percent as you can get it.

5. Next, gradually play with the speed of your workout until you come back up to 75 percent effort. By this we mean that you should experiment with different speeds until you get a nice feel for how fast you need to move to elicit the heart rate response you need.

Following this routine for the recommended period of weeks will greatly improve endurance and your overall fitness, too. Getting your heart rate to go up will take faster and longer pickups. The result is that you will cover more distance during the 20-minute workout. You also will enjoy a nice, safe improvement in your speed without risk of injury because, at the upper limit of 75 percent MHR, your pickups will always be aerobic and, therefore, free of lactic acid buildup in the muscles.

Fartlek is a Swedish word we translate as "speed play." After your first couple of workouts, you'll have a mental measure of the effort and be able to roller-coaster your heart rate up and down without too much difficulty. How long you take to work up to 75 percent and then coast down to 60 percent will be your choice. This option gives you a choice of a variety of movements. You can increase the effort to 75 percent quickly by going faster, recover to 60 percent slowly by gradually easing off the pace, or vice versa.

Fartlek workouts are a creative version of interval training without the rigorous repetitions of the same distance. It is a training system that can be used for the development of all four fitness components of endurance, stamina, economy, and speed.

The system originated in the 1930s and was made famous in the 1940s by Gunder Hagg and Arne Anderson, who took turns lowering the world record for the mile as they tried to break the barrier of the magic 4-minute mile. Hagg eventually got his time down to 4:01.4, where the record stood for nine years until Roger Bannister ran 3:59.4 in 1955.

LSD training, on the other hand, is all about consistency of pace and effort. Rather than roller-coasting your heart rate up and down, you simply maintain the same jog, or slow run, pace over a set period of time. As you work your way into shape, you start at the lower end of the intensity range (60 to 75 percent MHR) to maintain the same pace for the allotted time and distance. Your heart rate will gradually rise to 75 percent as the workout continues. As your fitness improves, you'll find it easier to train at a higher intensity with the same sense of effort, resulting in either more distance covered in the same amount of time or the same distance covered in less time.

A note of caution: Depending on the shape you're in, the opposite may happen. You may start out working too hard and reach your upper heart rate target in less than a New York minute. If so, then you'll have to spend your whole workout tapping the brakes to stay in this zone. It's best to keep in mind the advice of that great philosopher Walt Stack: "Go out slowly and then taper off."

LSD training is the natural follow-up to fartlek training. As you increase fitness through fartlek training, you will be able to hold your pickups close to and at 75 percent for longer and longer periods. Eventually, you will be able to complete the entire training session holding pace at 75 percent MHR with no need to slow down to keep your heart rate from creeping up over 75 percent. When you get to this point, you are ready to add LSD training to the mix. The LSD training will be done at a lower intensity to allow you to go longer, but the concept is the same: maintain an aerobic pace for the desired duration, gradually increasing that duration for greater endurance.

Another note of caution: To avoid overuse injuries, sports medicine specialists advise that the volume of work should increase only 10 to 15 percent per week. Obviously, caution needs to be exercised, but for a runner starting at 10 miles (16 km) per week, adding just 1 to 1.5 miles (1.6 to 2.4 km) over the week might be a little too conservative.

Duration of Workouts for Endurance Development

Ultimately, you will execute the workouts outlined in this chapter for longer periods of time. However, for an exercise session to provide enough stimulus to elicit a conditioning effect, it must last a minimum of 20 minutes. The number of times that you fartlek your heart rate up and down in your 60 to 75 percent effort zone depends on your level of general fitness. As you get stronger and fitter, it will gradually take longer to elevate your heart rate to your upper target and take less time to recover.

This 20-minute period may seem too short, and with the intensity so low, you may think that it is too easy. You may wonder whether you'll ever get in shape at this rate. But hold on. This is a very delicate period of adaptation. Your muscular system will get stronger rather quickly thanks to its good blood supply and may give you the impression that you're ready for bigger and better workouts. At the start of this period of getting into shape, you will probably experience some muscle stiffness and soreness. But, you'll find that you quickly get over those little aches and pains, and your engine will start adding horsepower. To avoid setbacks, we suggest that you follow a hard/easy pattern of workouts until you finish the recommended number of weeks appropriate for your circumstance.

Sample Base-Building Training Pattern

At its most elemental level, here's how a typical training plan begins and follows the classic pattern of hard/easy days. We use the word *hard* rather loosely here to refer to the days that you do the heart rate fartlek workouts. The rest of the days are easy, continuous activity at 60 to 65 percent MHR, or are totally off (because nothing is easier than a day off).

Please keep in mind as you study these samples that they are designed to demonstrate the principles involved and are not training programs. The sample training programs presented in the last chapters of the book contain the progressions in volume, intensity, and frequency that you would realistically expect to follow.

For weeks 1 and 2, follow this pattern:

- Hard days (Monday and Thursday): 20-minute heart rate fartlek at 60 to 75 percent MHR. The 20 minutes do not include slow, easy warm-up activity or a similar period for cooling down at less than 60 percent MHR.

- Easy days (Tuesday and Saturday): 20-minute recovery effort at a steady pace of 65 to 70 percent MHR. Follow the same warm-up and cool-down patterns as you used on the hard days.

- Off days (Wednesday, Friday, and Sunday): Take days off. These are complete rest days with no activity.

If you experience any aches or pains or feel you need more time to adjust to this routine, extend these workouts for another week or two. If you feel good and are ready and eager to advance to harder work, move on to the next pattern.

For weeks 3 and 4, follow this pattern:

- Hard days (Tuesday and Thursday): 20-minute heart rate fartlek at 60 to 75 percent MHR.
- Easy days (Monday and Friday): 25- to 30-minute recovery effort at 65 to 70 percent MHR.
- Long workout (Saturday): Begin to extend your continuous easy effort at 65 to 70 percent by making this workout 5 minutes longer than the time of your Monday and Friday workout each week until you reach 45 minutes.
- Off days (Wednesday and Sunday): Take these days off.

Keep repeating this pattern until you can do the heart rate fartlek workouts for 30 minutes by adding 3 to 5 minutes to them each week. Gauge your readiness to increase the length of the workouts by how your legs feel. Fartlek workouts are a rather artistic system of training that allows you the freedom to determine your own fate. One good rule of thumb to apply is the "three out of four" rule—every fourth week should be a shorter or lower-intensity recovery week.

Be very conservative about how fast you add more volume in these zones to give those connective tissues a chance to strengthen so you don't blow your transmission. One sign that you are ready to move on would be noting that your fitness level has improved to the point that the distance covered during the workouts has plateaued.

Once you are ready, move to the following plan for the next two to four weeks, adding the other endurance-building workout—long, slow distance, or LSD—to the pattern. Use nothing harder than 75 percent MHR on the LSD.

For the next two to four weeks, follow this pattern:

- Hard days (Tuesday and Saturday): 30 minutes of heart rate fartlek at 65 to 75 percent MHR.
- Hard days (Thursday and Sunday): 45 to 60 minutes of LSD at 60 to 75 percent MHR.
- Easy days (Monday and Wednesday): 30 to 45 minutes of recovery effort at 65 to 70 percent MHR.
- Off day (Friday): Take the day off to recover fully.

Start adding 5 minutes per workout to the time of your easy recovery days from the previous pattern. Work up to 45 minutes on Thursday and 60 minutes on Sunday.

During these weeks, the increased frequency of six sessions per week will result in your experiencing some days of accumulating fatigue in your working muscles. We've also increased the intensity of the heart rate fartlek by raising the lower limit of the recovery target heart rate from 60 to 65 percent MHR. This will make the workout harder by cutting down the recovery time. All that is due to our deliberate attempt to create a short-term chronic glycogen deficit in your muscles to stimulate the cells to use more fat as fuel. The easy days will allow you to recover, but you will also have to make a determined effort to slow down and take it easy on the recovery workouts. To be sure that you recover as much as possible, keep you upper target heart rate at just 70 percent. You'll notice that these workouts are definitely much harder, but still in the zone of low risk of injury.

If going so easy on your recovery days seems like punishment, keep this pearl of physiology in mind: The easier and more aerobic the workout, the more oxygen is present in the circulating blood. It is then available for the muscle to use so it can burn a higher percentage of its fuel from fat, thus sparing the carbohydrate you eat for conversion to glycogen.

Transition to Enhance Endurance

A consequence of lower-intensity, easier endurance development training is the less-than-complete strengthening of muscles, ligaments, and tendons. Another, by the very definition of aerobic work (no huffing and puffing allowed), is that your respiratory system's muscles are just beginning to get into good shape. Now it's time to move those parts of your body through a transition zone that will focus on the upper edge of your aerobic capacity. The extra effort and speed will put a little more stress on these systems and will prepare you for the strains of high-intensity anaerobic conditioning that will come when you move up the training triangle into the stamina, economy, and speed zones.

This transition work will be in the steady-state zone of 75 to 80 percent MHR. These two percentages are, respectively, right at the top of the aerobic zone and right at the bottom of the anaerobic zone. Workouts in this zone can put a modest stress on your respiratory system while you push your biomechanical system through bigger and faster ranges of motion.

To see what we mean, picture this example of someone making this transition from jogging and easy, low-intensity LSD running to steady-state running:

- On easy days, she's not just jogging with those little, bitty, mincing steps anymore or alternating easy strides for short fartlek pickups.
- She's running lightly and comfortably with a smoother, longer, but not full stride for extended periods of time.
- She's not breathing hard, but may have to talk in Hemingway sentences, which are much shorter than the Faulkner-style run-on sentences she used when jogging.
- She feels like she could run forever at this pace, which is close to what she would do if in shape to run for 10 to 13 miles (16 to 21 km).

Picture yourself doing your activity of choice at an effort comparable to this example, and then apply the following sample workout pattern to your sport.

Sample Endurance Enhancing Training Pattern

Earlier in this chapter we introduced the concept of hard/easy training by alternating days of light-intensity exercise with complete days off for full recovery. Granted, the days of easy workouts probably did not require much time for energy restoration. However, they were important for giving your legs time to build stronger muscles and tendons. As you climb up the training triangle to harder levels of effort, the recovery days become even more important. Effective recovery between steady-state hard days at 75 to 80 percent MHR demands that you keep your effort at 70 percent and lower on easy days. At this level of seriousness, you will still be working out on easy days with the emphasis on burning fat for fuel. Review the following workout pattern and then compare it with your endurance pattern. Picture yourself following these principles while pursuing the sport of your choice. The times in the following sample vary widely because of the differences in sports. See the chapter on your sport of interest for more appropriate workouts.

We assume that the long workout is on the weekend because most people have more time available on Saturday or Sunday. This example uses Sunday; if your long workout is on Saturday, just move everything back one day.

- Sunday: 45 to 90 minutes in the 65 to 75 percent MHR zone. Because of the length of this workout, even though the intensity is rather low, we consider it a hard day because of the amount of fuel burned.
- Monday and Wednesday: 20 to 45 minutes of easy recovery effort at 65 to 70 percent MHR.
- Tuesday and Saturday: 30 to 45 minutes of steady-state effort at 75 to 80 percent MHR. This includes 5 to 10 minutes at 60 to 70 percent to warm into the harder effort. Cool down with a few minutes of very easy, slow activity.
- Thursday: 5 to 10 minutes at 65 to 70 percent to warm up, then 15 to 20 minutes of heart rate fartlek, roller-coastering your heart rate up and down between 70 and 80 percent.
- Friday: Relax. You've worked long and hard, so take the day off.

After several weeks of this training pattern, you might want to do a time trial or jump into competition to see what kind of shape you are in. However, test or not, you will be ready to take your training up a notch to phase II and to the anaerobic threshold level of effort.

Maintenance of Aerobic Endurance

We offer a fairly generous target heart rate range of 60 to 75 percent to develop endurance. We offer the rather narrow but specific range of 75 to 80 percent MHR to enhance endurance. Two other target heart rate zones

Building Your Baseline, Trimming Your Waistline

If you're like us, you could be coming off the holiday season with a few extra pounds or kilograms and a bunch of missed workouts. However, in your haste to remedy the weight issue, you should literally slow down and consider the following points. First, although you might be concerned about body weight, doing the correct type of base training in the winter will more appropriately address this issue. Second, this time of year should be all about base building, or developing an aerobic foundation. Third, to do this, you must pick the correct low level of intensity. Not only will this help build your aerobic base, but it also will help with fat burning and weight control.

For simplicity, let's assume that the body burns carbohydrate and fat. At all times the body burns some combination of these two and never exclusively one or the other. We could further simplify this explanation by defining fat use as aerobic exercise and carbohydrate use as anaerobic exercise even though both contribute.

Assume we have two basic fiber types in skeletal muscle: fast-twitch and slow-twitch. They have different recruitment patterns that vary as a function of exercise intensity. Fast-twitch fibers are larger than slow-twitch fibers, and smaller fibers are always recruited first. We call this the size principle. As the intensity increases and more force is needed, more fast-twitch fibers are recruited. As force output or speed increases, you breathe more heavily at the same time that you need to produce more energy. In other words, you start to use more anaerobic energy or carbohydrate. The pattern goes like this: Increase the intensity, increase the fast-twitch recruitment; increase the fast-twitch recruitment, increase anaerobic metabolism; increase anaerobic metabolism, increase carbohydrate usage and decrease fat usage. So, to burn fat, you need to exercise slower.

Consider this: If you exercised at 85 to 90 percent MHR for 30 to 40 minutes, you would burn mostly carbohydrate. Carbohydrate is restored almost on a daily basis, which means that this approach causes very little fat weight loss. This is why many athletes exercise hard and yet do not lose weight and may, in fact, gain weight. The substrate (fat or carbohydrate) that is burned is pretty much a function of the oxygen available. The overall state of the cardiovascular and respiratory systems plays a large role in fuel economy. Increased aerobic fitness means increased fat burning. Therefore, you want to spend appropriate amounts of time developing your cardiorespiratory system at the right intensity. Here are some factors to consider:

- It takes 12 to 16 weeks to develop and deposit new blood vessels.
- The stimulus for developing and depositing new blood vessels is consistent aerobic stimulus lasting 40 minutes or more four or five times a week.
- The intensity must be such that it predominantly taxes the aerobic system and not the anaerobic system.
- The process takes time and patience.

In other words, aerobic base building and weight control require long periods of low-level, steady-state exercise, and the off-season is perfect for it.

Finally let's discuss the concept of exercise duration and a concept called oxygen deficit. Anytime metabolic intensity changes (you start to exercise or change the intensity during exercise), you'll notice a short period of discomfort or heavier breathing. This is because you have briefly moved from a dependence on aerobic metabolism to a

(continued)

Building Your Baseline   *(continued)*

dependence on anaerobic metabolism. After a few minutes, the respiratory and cardio-vascular systems catch up (reach a steady state), and this brief shortage of oxygen is corrected. This period of oxygen shortage is called the oxygen deficit, and it occurs at the beginning of exercise and with any changes in intensity.

What does all this mean? When you start to exercise, you experience an oxygen deficit that increases your dependence on anaerobic metabolism and carbohydrate. After 10 to 15 minutes, things settle down, and if the intensity is low enough, your dependence reverts back to fat. Even with this adjustment, it takes about 30 minutes to start using more fat than carbohydrate. This is why you must exercise steadily for 30 to 40 minutes for weight control. You can kill two birds with one stone by methodically designing your off-season program to focus on base building and by being patient.

within endurance range have useful purposes. They are known as *recovery zones*. Working out in these zones allow you to maintain endurance while your muscles rebuild and refresh themselves with new supplies of glycogen, that important source of energy used during longer and harder workouts.

In addition to using fat for fuel, muscles also burn a carbohydrate fuel known as glycogen. A good way to distinguish the two fuels is to think of fat as diesel fuel and glycogen as rocket fuel. Fat (diesel fuel) is a greasy, slow-burning source of energy that needs a lot of oxygen to be burned efficiently. Glycogen (rocket fuel) is highly volatile energy that can be burned in the absence of oxygen, although not efficiently for very long. Taking the car engine analogy a bit further, imagine that your muscles are the cylinders of an engine to which your carburetor sends both the gasoline and the oxygen to be ignited by electricity from the spark plug. The controlled explosion drives the piston up and down, creating movement just the way your muscles make your bones move back and forth. However, there is one very important difference between our imaginary engine and your body: your muscle cells are much more fuel efficient because they can burn two types of energy at the same time. Both diesel and rocket fuels are burned together so that the slow-burning fatty fuels are ignited by the hot-burning glycogen.

All this happens adequately in the 65 to 70 percent effort range because the slower paces at this lower level of intensity provide more oxygen, thus allowing more of the always-available free fatty acids to be burned, sparing the glycogen.

Of course, an even more effective recovery can be accomplished in the 60 to 65 percent effort zone, but at this level the pace becomes so slow that it takes the threat of arrest by the pace police to get anyone to take it that easy. Therefore, the only time we would recommend staying in this zone is the day before an important competition if you are one of those compulsive, obsessive athletes who worry about getting out of shape if they miss a day of training.

If you have become hooked on smart exercise and want to develop a higher level of fitness, the next chapters offer guidelines to follow in your quest for stamina, economy, and speed. Now it's time to follow the old adage: If you want to race faster, you have to train faster.

CHAPTER 6

Raising Anaerobic Threshold

Chapters 1 through 4 provided a background in heart rate response and measurement and the use of a heart rate monitor. Chapter 5 got you started on the path to good fitness with phase I base training. You also learned how to develop and enhance endurance by using low-intensity workouts that can greatly improve cardiovascular, respiratory, and muscle cell function. That path developed a great base of aerobic endurance, the platform that every serious athlete needs to build on.

As you push the effort up to greater than 80 percent MHR, you'll really start putting stronger muscles on your bones and wind in your sails. You will notice that phase II training, stamina training at 80 to 85 percent MHR, causes you to fail the all-important talk test. Even Hemingway's short, terse sentences will be too much. At best, as you concentrate on breathing, between huffs and puffs you might want to utter a "Yes" or a "No" or sputter a quick "Can't talk now!" to a question from a training partner. The third phase of training, economy training at 85 to 95 percent MHR, simply will take your breath away.

This chapter prepares you to maintain your goal pace for your desired duration by developing stamina and teaches the subtleties of pushing yourself toward athletically challenging peak performances by developing economy (your ability to go at race pace using the least amount of oxygen and energy), while mixing up your distances, speeds, and intensities.

By now we hope we've earned your confidence in our ability to improve your fitness. It will be even more important that you trust us as we develop your stamina, economy, and speed (to be covered in chapter 7). We all know that if you want to go faster, you must train faster, but we also know that risk of injuries from more extensive and intensive training is part of the game. By following our recommendations, you will decrease the risk of setbacks from injuries and illnesses. Get ready to swim, run, cycle, ski, row, or perform any activity you want, at a higher intensity. Now we pick up the pace.

Physiological Adaptations to Stamina (AT) Training

It is always important to understand why you are doing a certain type of training. In chapter 5 we provided some insight into what changes take place during endurance training and what you can expect from that level of training. These initial adaptations serve as the foundation for the adaptations that follow. The initial adaptations are arguably the most extensive; those that follow in later phases could be viewed more as refinement.

Adaptations to stamina training are numerous and include changes to the musculoskeletal, cardiorespiratory, and endocrine (hormonal) systems. The endocrine system was not so developed in the endurance phase. Adaptations in the musculoskeletal system arise from an increased contraction force over longer distances. During this phase of training, movement speed increases. This means that muscles contract at a slightly higher force causing greater changes in their overall strength and composition. This lays the groundwork for other biochemical changes that will take place in phases III and IV. This increased force of contraction causes an increased recruitment of the desirable fast-twitch fibers, which paves the way for faster speeds. Up until this point, except for the short fartlek pickups, most work has required only slow-twitch muscle fiber recruitment.

The cardiorespiratory system is enhanced further because it operates at a higher overall level for the duration of an exercise bout. Specifically, higher rates of respiration allow greater provision of oxygen and, very important, greater removal of carbon dioxide. Additionally, respiratory muscles move through greater ranges of motion at faster rates of contraction, which again lays the foundation for the heavier-intensity work to come in phases III and IV.

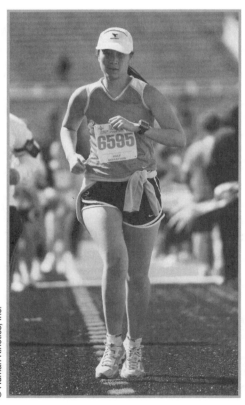

© Human Kinetics, Inc.

Smart training will prepare your body to maintain a consistent work rate over several miles so you finish strong.

Phase II also starts to introduce some subtle biochemical changes that relate to both energy usage and lactic acid tolerance. This increased work rate causes an initial increase in carbohydrate reliance, necessitating more structured rest and nutrition. Also, you will start to develop an increased capacity to tolerate lactic acid, allowing you to perform at higher work rates without undue discomfort.

The all-encompassing changes that take place in this phase permit the body to develop a consistent work rate that can be maintained over several miles or several hours. This is crucial because it indicates the body's ability to regulate temperature, maintain blood flow, remove waste products, and provide continuous energy resulting in the ability to maintain your higher work rate for longer periods.

The goals in phase II are to subtly increase the ability of all systems to function at a higher level with the ultimate goal of setting up for the higher-intensity work in phases III and IV. In fact, you could consider phase II an intermediary, or transition, step. Let's look at how to accomplish these goals.

Stamina Development

Now it's time to move your body through a transition zone that focuses on the anabolic (building) effects of anaerobic threshold (AT) exercise by putting a little more stress on the system. Although the obvious benefit to stamina training is the ability to maintain one's pace longer, this type of training is equally important in preparing you for the catabolic (tearing-down) strains of higher-intensity anaerobic conditioning that will come when you move from the phase II stamina stage on the training triangle into phase III economy workouts at 85 to 95 percent and, in chapter 7, into phase IV speed zones of 95 to 100 percent. For now, the focus is on increasing the top end of your aerobic system by training at or near your anaerobic, or lactate, threshold, the point at which your energy system moves in its reliance from aerobic to anaerobic energy production.

The term *anaerobic threshold* (AT) is widely used in a number of training environments. Coaches, athletes, and trainers commonly refer to AT as a focal point to determine the intensity of training. Consequently, much attention has been placed on the accurate measurement of AT and its interpretation for use in training programs. In the literature, several terms are used to denote this 80 to 85 percent zone, including *anaerobic threshold, lactate threshold*, and *ventilatory threshold*.

All of these terms refer to basically the same thing—that level of exercise at which a steady-state blood lactate concentration is no longer observed and it accumulates, creating a more acidic environment in the muscle. The lactate threshold explains several occurrences in muscle activity, and there are many theories for this increase in lactate. Lactate is a product of anaerobic metabolism when there is not enough oxygen to reduce it to a substance called acetyl-CoA; it occurs in greater amounts at high metabolic work rates because less oxygen is available. Thus, it appears to be intensity related. Other theorists suggest that a critical intensity and certain power output are required for lactate to accumulate. This power output can be met only by increased recruitment of fast-twitch fibers, which burn more carbohydrate and hence produce more lactate. These fast-twitch fibers are more anaerobic, which explains the increased lactate production.

Regardless of the specific intensity, lactate accumulation occurs at a non-linear rate that ultimately compromises muscle contraction. Thus, a person's fiber distribution may affect the anaerobic threshold. In addition, because increasing levels of lactate indicate higher levels of carbon dioxide, ventilation rates also increase as intensity increases. Thus we also see a nonlinear rise in ventilation (hence the term *ventilatory threshold*). The intensity of exercise is the primary determinant of lactate accumulation, and the higher the intensity, the greater the accumulation. Track events such as the 400- and 800-meter dash produce much higher lactate concentrations than the 3,000- or 10,000-meter run. Note that the body always produces lactate, and resting levels in trained athletes are typically between 1.5 and 2.0 mmol/L versus the suggested 4 mmol/L at which AT occurs.

Another very important issue needs to be addressed before proceeding. Anaerobic thresholds vary widely among individuals and sports. They also vary substantially within individuals, depending on fitness, throughout the conditioning process. Anaerobic thresholds can occur from 65 to 95 percent of maximum heart rate (MHR). Untrained people typically can hit anaerobic threshold at the low end of the heart rate range, whereas really well-trained people can work all the way up to 95 percent MHR before reaching anaerobic threshold.

Key Benefit of AT Training

The reason anaerobic threshold is important is that you can spend only a limited amount of time exercising above anaerobic threshold. Therefore, increasing anaerobic threshold allows you to exercise at a higher intensity for longer periods at a steady rate. Additionally, above the anaerobic threshold, glycogen becomes the primary fuel source, which means that you have a limited supply of energy.

Note that the value of anaerobic threshold training is not universally accepted. Measurement errors, individual variability, diet, and other factors can affect the outcome. Also, localized muscle action clearly influences lactate concentration in the muscle, which does not necessarily represent the amount of lactate in the body as a whole. Regardless, knowledge of the anaerobic threshold will ensure higher-intensity training that will allow you some measure of change in the cardiorespiratory response to a given workload. This simple approach will help you determine whether your performance times are improving. In all cases your success depends on your ability to monitor and evaluate your responses to a given workload.

Determining Your Anaerobic Threshold Heart Rate

How can you find out what your AT heart rate is? For absolute accuracy, you can go to a lab and pay for a test, but there are a few simple ways that will give you pretty decent numbers.

The first method is the talk test, and it's quick and easy. Plan a 30-minute run on flat ground (a track is ideal) with a friend you like to chat to. Start really slow and go at that pace for 5 minutes, all the time monitoring your heart rate while keeping up a lively conversation. After 5 minutes, increase your speed ever so slightly and continue monitoring and chatting. Repeat this procedure every 5 minutes until you notice that conversation is difficult to maintain; at this point you are around your AT.

The second method for determining your AT is a little more accurate. Actually, you do the same talk test, except this time you do it by yourself so you don't have to talk. The key is to monitor your heart rate very closely. Each time you increase your speed at the 5-minute mark, you'll notice that your heart rate increases for the first 60 to 90 seconds and then levels off. However, after you perform the third or fourth speed increase, you'll notice that your heart rate doesn't level off but instead keeps creeping up. The last level heart rate (also called steady state) you observed is a decent indicator of your AT. You can perform this procedure while biking, swimming, or rowing, as well.

Now that you have your AT heart rate, what does this number mean, and how do you use it? As you know, this heart rate indicates a threshold at which different adaptations occur depending on whether you are above it or below it. At this point, a simple guideline would be to say that while working in phases I and II, your heart rate is below AT, and then when you move to phases III and IV, your heart rate is above AT. In other words, use the AT heart rate as a check for your intensity in different phases. This will help ensure that you get the desired adaptations during each phase.

Your goal is to increase your AT over time with training. You should retest your AT about every eight weeks, and then reconfigure your intensities accordingly.

Transition to Stamina Training

One unfortunate side effect to all the endurance training covered in chapter 5 is that it won't really prepare you to compete in a race. You could run the race slowly at training pace, but if you run any faster, the resulting stiffness and soreness would not be worth it. This section explains two things that will help you overcome that handicap:

1. How to prepare to participate in events if your goal is simply to finish with a smile without concern about your place and time

2. How to prepare for the much harder, higher-intensity training required if your goal is to compete in events against the clock and other athletes

A primary objective of stamina training is to tax the respiratory system by going for longer periods of time. You want to improve your capacity so you won't get winded so easily. You want to be able to huff and puff and not go into terminal oxygen debt. All your other systems will also get in better shape, but stamina work is mostly about preparing for the next level of work and raising anaerobic threshold.

Following are general guidelines for determining your readiness to move from phase I (endurance) training to phase II (stamina) training:

- A steady and consistent 8 to 12 weeks of phase I training at least three times a week (shorter periods will work if the frequency is increased to five or six times per week)
- A noticeable decrease in the perceived effort of a 30-minute or more continuous effort at speeds (paces) the same as when you started
- A decrease in resting heart rate of 10 to 20 bpm (hard numbers are difficult to give here because people are so variable)
- A significant decrease of 5 to 7 bpm in heart rate response to moving at the rates, speeds, and paces you started with at the beginning of phase I training
- Faster rates, speeds, and paces at the same target heart rate
- Confidence that you can increase intensity without fear of injury or fatigue

If you have observed these changes, rest assured that your phase I training has prepared you to start pushing your workouts in the range of 80 to 85 percent MHR.

Training Techniques for Developing Stamina

Stamina training can be accomplished using several methods, but we will focus on three that target stamina and at the same time make effective use of a heart rate monitor. You can choose to use one method exclusively or combine methods, alternating among two or even all three within your training. Keep in mind that this discussion assumes that you warm up with easy activities in the 60 to 75 percent zone for 5 to 10 minutes and take a similar amount of time cooling down to reduce your heart rate to less than 60 percent.

- **Method 1:** Our version of heart rate fartlek can be adapted easily for stamina development. Expand the target heart rate zone offered in chapter 5, working up to 85 percent MHR and recovering to less than 70 percent MHR. During a 15- to 30-minute period, roller-coaster your heart rate up and down within this zone several times using your artistic sense to determine how hard to work (how fast to go) to get it into the 80 to 85 percent zone and how easy to take it (how slow to go) to recover to less than 70 percent.

- **Method 2:** A second way to improve AT and, therefore, stamina is tempo workouts, which we define as continuous efforts that last 15 to 30 minutes for the average athlete. Time ranges vary according to both fitness level and sport. More advanced athletes in sports that generate higher mileage (cyclists, for example) may extend this time period to 60 minutes but will rarely go beyond this because other challenges with nutrition and hydration start to become an issue. Start the workout with 5 to 10 minutes of easy to moderate effort at 60 to 70 percent to warm up. Increase the pace to reach 80 percent MHR. This allows you to start timing the AT period of the workout. Once at 80 percent, try a little harder to raise intensity until your heart rate gets into the upper level of your target zone at 85 percent. Once there, settle into the tempo of the workout. Make sure to back off the pace each time your heart rate monitor warns you that you're exceeding 85 percent.

• **Method 3:** Interval training is another effective technique for developing stamina. Thanks to the recovery intervals, interval training enables you to easily move faster and raise your heart rate quicker into your target zone of 80 to 85 percent because of the shorter periods or distances of your repeats. Simply divide the distance to be covered into shorter segments and follow each with a rest interval that allows your heart rate to recover to 70 percent or lower. For example, instead of a 20-minute tempo run, you run a mile three times, with intervals of jogging after each mile until your heart rate recovered. Because interval training for runners is almost always most conveniently done on a 400-meter track, a similar segment would be 1,600 meters with a 400-meter jog.

A more detailed explanation of the application of interval training appears later in this chapter in the section Sample Training Pattern to Improve Economy (page 82), which uses interval training as its sole training method. The principles presented there are also relevant here in terms of stamina interval training.

Although most coaches and athletes prefer tempo workouts that are uninterrupted periods of activity, near or at the 85 percent target to improve stamina, all three of these methods can be used to increase stamina. Each workout type requires faster speeds compared to phase I levels, regardless of whether you run, row, swim, bike, or whatever. The point is that you have to elevate your level of intensity (try harder), and that means going faster. With that said, there are specific benefits to each workout type.

Fartlek training is ideal for those whose personalities are on the artistic, creative, and philosophical edge and who are leery of the regimentation of interval training. It is also ideal for someone who prefers to just participate in events and finish smiling. By offering the choice of how quickly to elevate heart rate to the target of 85 percent, it could have the benefits of speed work. Fartlek training also works well for those who get impatient at running slowly all the time because it offers the option of routine increases in speed but without the stop-and-go nature of intervals.

Tempo workouts are good for swimmers, cyclists, runners, rowers, and cross-country skiers. They can greatly sharpen your sense of perceived exertion at anaerobic threshold paces. Because of the compact nature of tempo workouts, they often are more time efficient than either fartlek or interval workouts. They do tend to be psychologically more demanding because you have to maintain a higher intensity for periods of 20 to 30 minutes. With fartlek and interval training, the higher intensities are held for much shorter periods, usually less than 5 minutes.

Interval training in the stamina zone has the extra benefit of improving your sense of pace as you try to match pace and heart rate. Also, because you have a shorter period in which to elevate your heart rate, the pace, or speed, of the workout will be faster, thus developing a little bit of economy.

Sample AT Training Pattern to Improve Stamina

To maximize training effects, consider alternating techniques on your hard days. You'll get the benefit of some variety in your weekly pattern. This pattern uses two or all three of the training methods depending on your goals and fitness level.

We assume that your long workout will be on a weekend day because most people have more time available on Saturday or Sunday. This example uses Sunday; if your long, slow distance (LSD) workout is on Saturday, just move everything back one day. The times in the following sample vary widely to account for the differences in sports. See the chapter on your sport of interest for more appropriate workouts.

- Moderate day (Sunday): 45 to 90 minutes of LSD in the 65 to 75 percent MHR zone. This workout, depending on its length, can either maintain or enhance endurance. Because of the length, even though the intensity is rather low, we consider it a moderate to hard day because of the amount of fuel you'll burn.

- Easy days (Monday and Wednesday): 20 to 45 minutes of easy recovery effort at 65 to 70 percent MHR. This slow, easy effort will allow you to spare the carbohydrate you eat and give you the time needed to convert it into glycogen. Instead you'll burn fat for your primary energy source.

- Hard day (Tuesday): 15 to 30 minutes of nonstop tempo training at 80 to 85 percent MHR. This doesn't include a 5- to 10-minute warm-up and the few minutes of transition to 80 percent. Cool down with a few minutes of very easy, slow activity.

- Hard day (Thursday): After warming up, do a more moderate but longer steady-state workout at 75 to 80 percent for 45 to 60 minutes. If you are an advanced athletes who can handle three hard workouts per week, you could substitute a heart rate fartlek workout at 80 to 85 percent MHR; however, be very careful because the introduction of hard workouts increases the risk of overtraining and injury. Be very cautious about moving to three hard sessions a week.

- Off day (Friday): Relax. You've worked long and hard, so take the day off.
- Easy to moderate day (Saturday): Knowing that you will go for a long, moderate workout tomorrow, you might just run another easy effort like the one you do on Monday and Wednesday. Or, after warming up, you could do an interval workout of three 6-minute bouts at 80 percent MHR with 3 minutes of easy recovery activity to bring your heart rate down to less than 70 percent.

Repeat this pattern for the next three or four weeks. As a general rule, do not add or move up to a higher-intensity workout until you have performed the same workouts at the same intensity for two to four weeks.

Please note: It is easy to turn AT workouts into something harder than appropriate. Letting the effort slip into the economy zone above 85 percent can be fatal to your progress. If your heart rate starts to go over that limit, back off the effort, the pace, the stroke rate, pedal speed, or whatever.

It is extremely important that you buy into the notion that training for aerobically oriented athletic performances is generally not about being mentally tough and therefore pushing yourself into exhaustive degrees of fatigue. Yes, there is a time and place for workouts that drop you to your knees or make you almost fall off your bike. We'll get to those much later. Training with a heart rate monitor and with our guidelines is about learning the art of finesse. Finesse is finding the fine line of hitting your target for the day and not pushing over it. Finesse leads to training consistency because you leave your workout feeling exhilarated and stimulated, not riddled with such deep levels of fatigue that you have to drag yourself to the shower and then crash onto the couch for a nap. These guidelines create training that is perfectly tailored to your current level of fitness as well as your goal. It's all to answer the "What about me?" question.

Pushing beyond your target zones makes you just like everyone else who mistakenly thinks that harder is better. You don't have to outwork your competition. You just have to outsmart them.

A seeming paradox needs explanation at this point. A poorly appreciated fact about AT training is that you will get faster at the same level of perceived exertion. This is true because your AT and the actual heart rate at which it occurs are highly fluid. Depending on your current level of fitness, you can experience AT from 65 to 95 percent of MHR. It may seem nutty for us to be emphasizing that stamina is developed at 80 to 85 percent in phase II, but you can improve AT in every phase of training. Yes, over the course of your training, your heart rate at your AT will get higher, but the ironic thing is that you won't notice any increase in the effort because you will always start huffing and puffing at your AT. You'll simply be getting in better shape.

Here's the really good news: This automatically results in going faster. Once you are in your AT zone, you will feel no desire to talk. The effort should feel uncomfortable, yet sustainable for the core period you've picked for your workout. Within minutes of finishing your cool-down, you should experience a strong feeling of bounce in your walk. Once you are in phase II, your workouts in this wonderfully productive 80 to 85 percent zone do not allow for much lactic acid buildup, so your muscles won't tighten and then get strained, stretched, and torn. If you finessed the workout, you should not feel stiff and sore the day after.

The next sections cover the guidelines for transitioning to economy training, and in the next chapter we give more definitive guidelines for when to move to higher-intensity interval training. It's now time to deliberately push into the next zone of training and take a closer look at the training goal of economy development.

Physiological Adaptations to Economy Training

As you move up the training triangle to the next level of conditioning, your fitness will improve from the higher-stress workouts at 85 to 95 percent MHR. The following adaptations will happen with the right stimulus:

- Another improvement in maximum oxygen uptake ($\dot{V}O_2max$) as stress on the respiratory system increases the strength of the intercostal and diaphragm muscles.
- The size of the capillary bed in the muscles increases in response to the presence of more lactic acid. This facilitates greater blood flow in and out of the muscle allowing more delivery of oxygen and greater removal of waste products.
- Flexibility improves as the limbs work through greater ranges of movement.
- Strength increases as greater effort recruits more muscle fibers, especially fast-twitch fibers.
- Coordination among mind, nerves, and muscles improves because more concentration is required at these higher intensities.
- Stimulation of the pituitary gland increases the release of human growth hormone promoting greater muscle development response.

One unfortunate side effect may be a decrease in libido as a result of the high stresses of heavy training. Hey, you can't have it all.

Economy Development

We like to define the component of fitness we call economy as the capacity to maintain race pace while the muscles use the least amount of oxygen and energy possible. Training fast and hard enough to reach the heart rate zone of 85 to 95 percent develops stronger, bigger muscles. In other words, you spread the load across the muscle fibers and recruit more muscle fibers to reduce the load on individual fibers. Think of it like a car engine that is built to go 120 miles per hour (193 km/h). At this top speed, the car would get lousy gas mileage and be quite costly to drive. But at a speed limit of 65 miles per hour (104 km/h), with much better gas mileage, the car becomes more economical to operate.

It might help to make a distinction between *efficiency* and *economy*, two words that people have a tendency to use interchangeably. We like to relate efficiency to the biomechanics of the body's movements, whereas economy refers more to the use of oxygen and the fuels that the body uses to move. Again, with our car analogy, correcting the wheel alignment of a car that pulls to the right when your hands are off the steering wheel eliminates inefficient movement and thus makes it more economical to drive. Improving your form by working on your biomechanics can have the same result. By training at faster than goal paces to build a bigger engine, less

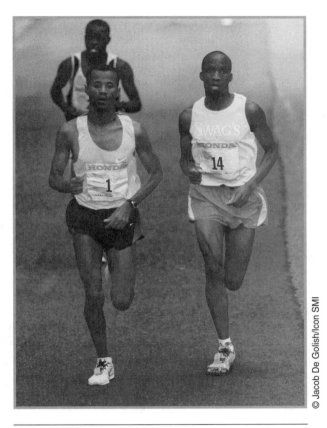

Training at higher intensities than will be needed in competitive conditions makes the body work more economically during races. The body will require less fuel and oxygen to maintain race pace and delay fatigue.

© Jacob De Golish/Icon SMI

fuel and oxygen will be needed at the early, submaximum paces of a race. This will help save fuel supplies, anaerobic or carbohydrate, and delay the onset of fatigue.

Transition to Enhancing Economy

The economy phase of training increases the focus on the catabolic effects of highly anaerobic exercise due to the prolonged and elevated stress on your systems. Ultimately training in the economy phase causes some muscle breakdown. Although there are obvious physical benefits from economy training, there is a psychological one as well. You will experience the agony and pain of deep fatigue from oxygen deprivation. You will find out how the big bad wolf got tough enough to huff and puff until he blew the house down. In short, you'll develop some mental toughness.

Economy workouts are equally important in preparing you for even riskier catabolic strains of the higher-intensity anaerobic conditioning that will come when you move from phase III of the training triangle into phase IV (speed) workouts at 95 to 100 percent MHR in chapter 7. For now, the focus is on teaching your body to deal with loads of lactic acid that accumulate at highly anaerobic efforts.

The general guidelines for determining your readiness to move from phase II (stamina) training to phase III (economy) training are as follows:

- A steady and consistent two to four weeks of phase II training in the 80 to 85 percent zone
- No noticeable change in the perceived effort at AT even while going at faster speeds and at a higher heart rate
- A significant decrease of 5 to 7 bpm in the heart rate response when moving at the same rates, paces, and speeds of your first workouts
- Faster speeds, paces, and rates at all of the original heart rate training zones
- Confidence that you can increase intensity without fear of injury or fatigue

Most important, measuring your current fitness level by competing in a few races will let you know when you are ready to move up to a higher level of training. Wanting to beat the clock or the pants off a rival is a sure sign that you're ready for higher-intensity work.

Activities for Enhancing Economy

Once you have two to four weeks or so of stamina training under your belt, you are ready to add economy training to the mix. Our favorite training tool for moving from one training zone to the next is good old heart rate fartlek. Following the same pattern of daily workouts (running, cycling, or cross-country skiing) that you used in the section on stamina training, you can make your hard days even harder by going up hills long enough to raise your heart rate to 95 percent MHR. If you are a swimmer, you can increase drag by wearing a drag suit or doing harness work. If you are a rower, you can increase the drag factor on the rowing ergometer or increase your stroke rate on the water. Recovery on the downhills and flats should be slow enough to bring your heart rate down to less than 70 percent. Other choices of activities on flat surfaces would have to be done fast enough to achieve the same target heart rate.

A typical heart rate fartlek session should include several of these harder efforts lasting from 20 to 30 seconds up to a few minutes over the course of a 30- to 45-minute session.

Although we like the easy adaptability of fartlek workouts, probably the most effective and popular training system for developing economy is interval training—and it is especially conducive to heart rate monitoring. The following discussion may seem like more information than you need, but please be patient while you carefully study how we blend heart rate zone workouts, and then see how you can adapt them to interval training.

Consider the example of Lancetta, a cyclist who needs to develop her economy, her body's ability to use the least amount of oxygen and energy at race pace. Let's say that to win a 20-mile (32 km) cycling time trial race, Lancetta will need to average 20 miles per hour (32 km/h). Realizing she probably can't ride 20 miles every day at her race pace without trashing herself, she decides to break the distance into smaller segments of 2 miles (3 km). She'll do multiple segments of them in a single session. Lancetta guesses that if she rode just 2 miles at a time with a short break between them to recover her wind and energy, she could probably average 24 or even 25 miles per hour (39 or 40 km/h) for each 2-mile repeat. Then later, by slowing down to 20 miles per hour (32 km/h), she might be able to ride the whole 20 miles at her goal of 20 miles per hour without the rest intervals and thus win the race. Sure enough, by working the shorter segments with intervals of rest between them, she could practice covering her goal distance.

But how would Lancetta know if the workout of ten 2-mile (3 km) segments at 25 miles per hour (40 km/h) was too hard and if it might quickly result in training herself into the ground? Or what if it felt so easy that she were tempted to try more repeats of the 2-mile distance? Should she? We'll get to the answers soon, but first we will discuss what she is trying to do.

As you read the scenario, we hope you noticed the frequent use of the word *interval*. Yes, we are talking about interval training, the most effective and popular training system ever designed. You've probably noticed that the word *interval* refers to the recovery period between repeated high-intensity efforts. We bring this up because of the imprecise use of language in both the lab and the locker room. Your monitoring of this period of recovery between high-quality efforts for fairly short periods of time means that you will be counting and monitoring your declining heart rate during the interval of recovery time. Often the word *interval* is used to refer to the distance or time to be repeated at the higher intensity, and the period of recovery is given some other term, but not here! This is important because we are offering you a valid, reliable, scientific method of answering the "What about me?" question.

If you accept that every workout is an experiment, you'll have the beginning of your answer. If you believe us when we say that every experiment is simply made up of givens and a variable, you will be closer to your answer. If you trust us when we explain that the variable must measure something that you are trying to find out about yourself, and that the givens can't change during the experiment, then you can easily understand that the beauty of interval training is the whole answer. Best of all, it's the perfect use of a heart rate monitor because it measures your response to the givens and the variable. Maybe now you can see how this formula for interval workouts—number of repeats multiplied by the distance to be repeated in a target time with an interval of activity to allow recovery—came to be so ubiquitous.

Let's go back to Lancetta's interval training session to see how this works when someone does not use the experimental format that led to the invention of the interval training system. At this phase of her training, Lancetta's goal is to improve her economy. Lancetta does what every athlete or coach must do to design an interval workout: she arbitrarily divides the total distance into shorter segments. There is nothing particularly special about 2 miles (3 km); she could have picked 1 mile (1.6 km) to repeat. It doesn't really matter as long as it is short enough for her to maintain her intensity level of 85 to 95 percent for as much of the distance as possible. She has just picked something short enough that she is sure she can ride it at a pace significantly faster than race pace. Next, Lancetta decides to try covering the total distance of her goal race, 20 miles (32 km). That, of course, means that she has to ride 10 times the 2 miles at the given speed of 25 miles per hour (40 km/h). To be sure that she can keep this up, she has to decide arbitrarily how long to rest between the repeats to get her heart rate back down to less than 70 percent. She hopes that riding a slow mile will be enough. This, then, is the interval formula for her workout:

10 × 2 miles at 25 mph with an easy, slow 10 mph mile interval of recovery

What happens if she can't meet these criteria (10 repeats of 2 miles at 25 mph) during the workout? She may find that her workout is so hard that she can't do all 10 repeats, can't maintain 25 miles per hour (40 km/h) for all 10 repeats, can't recover during just 1 easy mile (1.6 km) and needs 2 miles (3.2 km), or meets all the criteria but only at an exhaustive, all-out 100 percent effort that is inappropriate for a practice day.

If she finds she requires an exhaustive 100 percent effort to meet the criteria, Lancetta may be proud that she had the guts to tough it out while probably not realizing that she is risking her health or overall training adaptation. If she finds any of the first three results, our guess is that she will feel like a failure. Regardless, she is not happy because it is apparent that she is not in the shape she thought she was or that she just had a bad day or couldn't cope with weather conditions. We all appreciate that an unsuccessful workout certainly does not build confidence.

Ironically, at this phase of training for a serious athlete, the problem is seldom the athlete's fitness, ability, or mental toughness. The usual problem is a workout that offers only givens without a variable. This leaves no wiggle room for finding reasons why things didn't work. When we analyze Lancetta's workout, we see that she needed three givens and one variable to truly measure what was happening. She didn't know that effort is the answer. How will she know if 25 miles per hour (40 km/h) is too hard or too easy? How will she know if she will be ready to go again after a slow 1-mile (1.6 km) recovery ride? Is 20 miles (32 km) too much or too little? To answer those questions, we first have to review the objective of Lancetta's workout. Along her trip up the training triangle through the four phases of training, every level of effort has to have a conditioning effect.

Her goal at this point of phase III conditioning is to improve her economy, and that requires an effort in the 85 to 95 percent zone of MHR. Therefore, the design of the workout must start with the assumption that the combination of the speed and the length of the distance to be repeated will bring her heart rate into the goal zone. With target heart rate now a given, and knowing that she wants to ride segments of 2 miles (3.2 km), the distance to be repeated also becomes a given. With the recovery interval planned to be 1 mile (1.6 km) at 10 miles per hour (16 km/h), that's another given. Therefore, on this day, her speed must be the variable.

Now that we know what the variable is, the formula for her interval workout can follow the experimental format, and we can fill in the details for the givens. Her givens are the number of repeats, the distance to ride, and length of the interval, so what she needs to know is whether the pace is correct. With Lancetta's measured MHR at 181 bpm, her target heart rate zone at 85 to 95 percent is 164 to 171 bpm. The workout, then, looks like this:

> 10 × 2 miles at (?) mph at HR 164 to 171 bpm with a recovery interval of 1 mile at 10 mph.

The question is, How fast will she need to ride to achieve the proper effort? If Lancetta cannot manage a speed over 20 miles per hour (32 km/h) without exceeding her upper heart rate limit, then she clearly is not ready to win the race. If she manages 25 miles per hour (40 km/h), she is probably ready to race right away. If she goes even faster for the whole workout, she can change her goal and maybe consider going pro.

If she does fall short, more time spent in this phase will allow her to get in better shape as she tries this workout again. After a few weeks, her improved speed should bring her pace up to the goal of 25 miles per hour (40 km/h). At that point, she should be able to slow down to her goal pace of 20 miles per hour (32 km/h) and go the whole 20 miles (32 km) without the recovery intervals. The benefit of this combination of experimental format and heart rate monitoring is that Lancetta repeats the same workout each week and exquisitely tracks the progress of her improved fitness. At the same effort, she gets faster. Bear in mind that she is always using heart rate as her effort guidance system.

You may have realized by now that this format has lots of potential for improving other levels of fitness. We could improve stamina by featuring longer repeats at a lower intensity:

> (?) × 5 miles at 20 mph with an interval of 1 mile at 10 mph

We could also add Lancetta's target heart rate at 80 to 85 percent and then the experiment looks like this:

> (?) × 5 miles at 20 mph at 145 to 164 bpm with 1 mile at 10 mph

In this scenario, Lancetta finds out how prepared she is to sustain her goal pace. If she can do only one or two rides without exceeding 164 bpm, she needs to spend a couple of weeks doing this workout until her stamina improves.

Chapter 7 looks ahead to the end of the season when Lancetta needs to be at her peak; at that point she will need to improve her power and lactic acid tolerance. Then she could do a much higher-intensity workout that uses the recovery interval as the variable.

Sample Training Pattern to Improve Economy

For variety and to maximize the training effects, this pattern for improving economy includes three different workouts for hard days. We assume that your long workout will be on a weekend because most people have more time on Saturday or Sunday. This example uses Sunday; if your long workout is on Saturday, just move everything back one day. The times in this sample have wide ranges to account for the differences in sports. See the chapter on your sport of interest for more appropriate workouts.

- Hard day (Sunday): 60 to 90 minutes of long, slow distance (LSD) at 60 to 75 percent MHR
- Easy days (Monday and Friday): 20 to 30 minutes of easy recovery effort at 65 to 70 percent MHR
- Hard day (Tuesday): 30-minute heart rate fartlek at 70 to 95 percent MHR
- Off day (Wednesday): Take the day off.
- Hard day (Thursday): 12 × 400 m at 90 to 95 percent MHR with rest interval to less than 70 percent MHR
- Moderate day (Saturday): 20 to 30 minutes of moderate steady-state effort at 75 to 80 percent MHR

Training at these high intensities requires careful attention to recovery days. Anyone can train hard, but smart athletes also know when to take it easy. Going slowly enough in the easy recovery zones is a challenge that requires self-discipline. Almost every athlete we know has complained about how hard it is to go slowly enough to stay in such low recovery heart rate zones. However, without full, complete recovery, you can quickly become overtrained or get sick or hurt.

Ironically, you will also need a great deal of self-discipline to avoid doing the first part of an interval workout too fast. When you're fresh and frisky at the start of the workout (just like you would feel on race day), it's very easy to develop the bad habit of going out too fast and hence too hard. Have you had the experience of starting too fast? Most of us have. After all, who can't push the pace up to 95 percent or more when they feel good?

When you start too fast, you soon learn the frustration of positive splits. Those are times for the last half or quarter of the race that are slower than those for the first section. Being passed at the end of a race because you shot your wad at the start is more than embarrassing; it's highly discouraging. If you're feeling sorry for yourself, it's easy to give up and slow down even more.

Unfortunately, interval training offers just that temptation. You need to realize that workouts are supposed to duplicate racing conditions. You want to do in practice what you need to do in a race: start the repeats by holding back. There is nothing wrong with going slow and easy at the start. It just means that you'll have the energy to go faster at the end.

To this end, expect to reach just the lower end of your target heart rate zone during the end of the first third or fourth of your full workout. As you continue through the workout, you should not have much trouble hitting the upper limit. In fact, be sure not to exceed it. That would make the workout too much like true speed work and could cause you to peak too soon. We get into that intensity of training in chapter 7.

An approach to ensure that you do not go too fast at first is to create subsplits within your work piece that allow you to gauge your pace halfway through the piece as opposed to at the end only. For example, let's say you are doing 800-meter repeats at a 3:30 pace. You could split this further into 200-meter and 400-meter subsplits. Your 400-meter subsplits would be 1:45, and your 200-meter subsplits would be 0:52 to 0:53. If you go through the first 200 meters at 0:46, you can adjust immediately instead of adjusting through dying over the last 200 to 300 meters.

At this time, your fitness level has improved to competitive levels and you should be enjoying steady improvements in your personal records (PRs). You have increased your efforts up to 95 percent MHR and have lived to tell about those feats of athletic daring. The key to surviving without injury or illness from overtraining is found on your recovery days of easy, slow, low-intensity work at highly aerobic levels of less than 70 percent MHR. The standard for open-class athletes is one recovery day for every hard day. For older athletes or those with more modest talent, it may be wise to take two or even three easy days in row.

In the next chapter about speed training, you'll learn the art and science of peaking for the end of the season and championship performances. Those workouts require both longer periods of recovery during workouts and between them. We wish you many happy heartbeats!

CHAPTER 7

Boosting Speed and Power

Hang on to your hat, tie your trunks tighter, and check your brakes. You are entering the fourth, and last, phase of training. You're about to do workouts that will bring you to the peak of your physical capacities. You'll be able to perform personal feats at your all-time best. To do so, we need to expand your understanding of speed by also introducing its close cousin, power.

In chapter 5 we suggested a target zone of less than 75 percent MHR (maximum heart rate) to initially improve endurance, a zone of 75 to 80 percent to enhance it, and a zone of 65 to 70 percent (or even 60 to 65 percent) to maintain it. Endurance training lays the foundation for higher-intensity work and also helps the body recover from it. Chapter 6 discussed improving stamina by upping the effort to 80 to 85 percent while training at anaerobic threshold. Then we showed you how to significantly increase your pace by working hard enough to exceed your anaerobic threshold (85 to 95 percent MHR) to develop your economy. After taking you progressively through the first three phases of training, we are now set to discuss the components of athletic capacity developed at 95 to 100 percent MHR: speed and power.

The terms *speed* and *power* are often are used interchangeably, but they are, in fact, very different. What is sometimes confusing is that both power and speed training occur within the same heart rate zone of 95 to 100 percent. However, speed development can occur at less than 95 percent MHR, whereas power training takes place only in the 95 to 100 percent zone and is, quite simply, maximum effort. Power training is explosive movement requiring all-out effort, whereas speed can improve across a range of submaximum heart rate zones. In other words, power training occurs at a higher intensity (maximum intensity). A quick example: An interval workout of 400-meter repeats would be speed training, whereas 40-meter sprints would be power training. Many athletes do power and speed work in the same exercise session. We'll have some examples of these workouts later in the chapter.

One further point of interest is that power training helps with speed, but the reverse is not as likely to happen—speed training won't necessarily help with power. To an endurance athlete, speed is more important than power. Endurance events are won by high average speeds not by intermittent bouts of power. Speed work can be both aerobic and anaerobic; power is almost exclusively anaerobic. Understanding the difference between these two components will help ensure that you design your training program adequately.

This chapter explains how to develop both speed and power, because doing so will inevitably allow you to run or bike or row at a faster average speed over your race distance. To keep the distinction between the two components clear, you can assume that power training requires an all-out effort lasting less than 10 seconds, whereas speed work may last 10 seconds to 10 minutes. Think back to the 400-meter and 40-meter example.

One area of potential confusion here relates to the heart rate response seen in both power and speed training. Interestingly, both methods of training, albeit different, usually have the same result—the heart rate at the end of the exercise bout is the same for both. The difference lies in the fact that, in power training, the heart rate response is more immediate, whereas in speed work, heart rate rises over the length of the exercise bout, reaching its highest only at the end.

You may have to do several repeats during either of these types of workouts to reach your true MHR. For example, if sprinting uphill for only 10 seconds is today's workout, you may have to perform several sprints to achieve a true MHR. Your immediate heart rate at the conclusion of a single repetition of a power workout might be surprisingly low. This is explained by the fact that sprint-type exercise occurs in a short period of time and is over before your heart rate catches up with the intense oxygen debt that was created. Therefore, you have to keep watching your heart rate monitor to see how high it spikes as you start your recovery interval. Even then, your heart rate may fall short of the 95 to 100 percent zone. If so, don't worry; just be sure that you still take every minute of a full recovery until your heart rate drops to less than 60 percent MHR, and that you continue with maximum efforts during your power repeats.

Power relates to your ability to do work over time, but also to how rapidly you can produce force, or in fitness jargon, accelerate and turn on the afterburners. More powerful people do things more quickly. Although power is not a large component in endurance training, it is needed. A cyclist climbing a hill, sprinting to the finish, or chasing a breakaway attempt requires power. A runner putting in a final kick for the finish line or maintaining speed on a hill needs power. Therefore, you need to include power work in your training. That's why we have it as the final phase.

Keep in mind that workouts mirror your heart rate response in a race; when you are fresh at the beginning, it is easier to work. Thus, your heart rate may be surprisingly lower than you'd expect. Your breathing may be as hard as it can be, but your heart rate may lag behind either early in the workout, at the end of short repeats, or both.

Before we offer some sample programs, let's take a look at some very important background information. Different types of training affect your muscles in different ways. Some build up muscle (anabolic); others break down muscle and fat (catabolic). Some types of exercise cause a mix of anabolic and catabolic responses. That's why, when you initially start an exercise program, you see some muscle buildup and some fat breakdown. However, you can also experience muscle breakdown even at low intensity. Enough long, slow endurance work at modest intensities of 75 to 80 percent MHR for the longer durations required for marathons and Iron

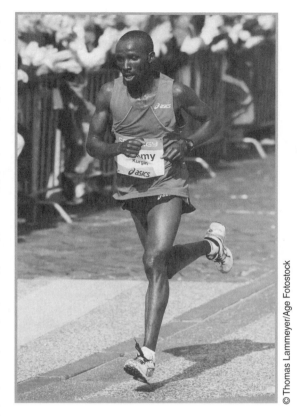

© Thomas Lammeyer/Age Fotostock

A runner needs power to make that final kick at the finish line.

Man triathlons, for example, can lead to muscle catabolism and therefore must be carefully monitored. In fact, athletes in these events often demonstrate low body weight because of both low body fat and less muscle mass.

All things considered, training at and below your anaerobic threshold is considered to have an anabolic effect initially on muscles. For that reason, it is not very risky. (However, even economy work at 85 to 95 percent MHR can have an unhealthy catabolic effect on your muscles, especially if the sessions are longer than 60 minutes.) Speed and power training in the 95 to 100 percent zone of MHR, the final category of fitness activity, is even harder on your body and must be carefully balanced with appropriate rest and nutrition. This is one reason you can run slowly six or seven days a week, but should do speed and power training only one or two days a week. Workouts at this level are needed to develop full sprint speed and lactic acid tolerance, both of which are necessary to bring you to peak performance capacity. You will definitely feel the burn as you add speed and power training to those last few weeks of workouts before your championship season.

Physiological Adaptations to Speed and Power Training

The movement into power and speed training signifies somewhat your readiness to do battle. You have gone through the slogging of marching and setting up the base. What you need to do now is fine-tune the engine and then let 'er rip. But just a little more patience is needed. Throughout phases I through III, you went through a steady increase in speed that was controllable, manageable, and above all, safe. In this last phase, you are going to be moving at full throttle, and you should be here only if you are confident that you have appropriately developed through the previous phases. We'll get more into the details of gauging your readiness later. For now, let's look at the final physiological adjustments and adaptations that, together with the three phases of foundation work, blend to create that well-oiled machine that will tick over at a nice high-energy rate while maintaining perfect form and function.

Phases I and II created mostly cardiorespiratory adaptations. Phase III created more biochemical adaptations on top of additional cardiovascular adaptations. In phase IV you are going to top off those biochemical adaptations to enhance both the cardiovascular and respiratory systems and ultimately improve total fitness and performance. Here are the adaptations you can expect:

- Faster recovery from high-intensity sessions
- Marked increases in acceleration and top speed
- Improved muscle biochemistry allowing greater tolerance and removal of metabolic waste products such as lactic acid
- Improved neural function and recruitment of both fast- and slow-twitch fibers
- Improved energy production rates and improved storage of glycogen
- Improved mechanics and form
- Greater mobility and flexibility through the greater ranges of movement required at faster speeds
- Slight increases in strength from the higher-intensity work and greater recruitment of fast-twitch muscle fiber
- Improved mood state from a reduction in total volume
- Decrease in muscle soreness from a reduction in total volume
- Improved ventilatory function from the higher ventilatory rates experienced during maximal work
- Improved performance

We do need to add one more adaptation, but it is a more psychological one. In phase IV, you may experience further increases in mental toughness as a result of repeated exposure to high-intensity, maximum-exertion work. Just as the body learns to tolerate higher levels of lactic acid, so also will the mind learn to tell the body to relax, keep going, and not give up when all the muscles are screaming for relief. Even though you may actually be slowing down as you near the finish line, speed and power training help you learn to not tighten up your muscles in an attempt to try even harder. This could be called the art of dying as your muscles tighten and you slow down gracefully at the slowest rate possible. Sometimes we like to say, "Yes, you'll be crawling, but you just have to crawl faster than the next guy." Speed work not only helps you get faster, but it also helps you stay fast longer. Talk about mental toughness. Do speed and power training, and you'll have it in spades.

Collectively, these final adaptations will put you in a position to perform optimally. At this point you will really be enjoying your exercise and clearly see your results. Your body will have toned up; you'll look lean and move fast (hopefully) and, with the correct nutrition, achieve your goal.

Speed and Power Development

You must progress slowly over the course of your peaking weeks to avoid injury. Your mental well-being may depend on staying healthy and avoiding the training room. That's why we advise slow progressions through all phases of training. The challenge at these risky levels is to carefully mix these high-intensity workouts with smaller volumes of work while maximizing the recovery intervals during the workouts and from one speed and power workout to the next.

Interestingly, this brings us back to the most important concept in this book—that effort is the answer and that you can effectively measure that effort with your heart rate monitor. Granted, learning to gauge your pace is an important skill and a very valid benefit of training, but measuring the difficulty or ease of your work effort and the quality of your recovery periods is the best way to guarantee the perfect adaptations you seek for your body.

You can pick a pace or rate of movement for your workout, but only by measuring how hard or easy it is will you know whether you picked properly. This is the feedback you want from your heart rate monitor. It is always trying to help you answer the vital "What about me?" question.

The best way to drive this point home and demonstrate what we mean by monitoring your effort is to offer typical examples of real-life training situations in which athletes use speed training to improve their overall endurance. Our examples bring together all the concepts of the book so you can anticipate the design of the sample training programs offered in later chapters. We offer a running example and a cycling example, both of which provide detail about strategy and how to put things together.

Our first example is of a session designed to improve overall speed. The workout includes both speed and power components. Table 7.1 identifies those workouts that are speed and those that are power. The split times selected for the running example are for a short-distance runner who can currently run a 5:30 mile.

TABLE 7.1 Sample Speed and Power Workout for a Short-Distance Runner

Piece	Split time	Rest interval	Focus	Percent MHR*
Warm-up	10:00			<75% MHR
2 × 800 m	2:30	<65% MHR	Speed	>95% MHR
3 × 400 m	0:65	<65% MHR	Speed	>95% MHR
4 × 75 m	Max effort	<60% MHR	Power	>95% MHR
5 × 40 m	Max effort	<60% MHR	Power	>95% MHR
Cool-down	5:00			<75% MHR

*Heart rates less than 95 percent may extend all the way to 100 percent. This can occur for both speed and power training.

This high-intensity interval workout balances the fast, hard efforts with plenty of recovery time between repeats. It covers a fairly short distance of just 3,300 meters, but offers lots of time of very low-intensity activities such as jogging or even walking to guarantee the clearing of oxygen debts and lactic acid accumulations. (Additional pieces can be added as the runner gets fitter and faster.) The split times should be fast enough for a runner in shape to run a 5:30 mile to raise heart rate to the goal of 95 percent or more. If the pace is too slow and fails to get the runner's heart rate to 95 percent or more, the runner could go faster, but we do not recommend starting the next repeats without achieving the desired recovery interval target heart rate.

In this interval session, the speed increases as the distance decreases. When the distance drops to 75 meters and then again to 40 meters, both of these pieces are performed at maximum sprint pace to develop power. The 800-meter and 400-meter pieces are not done at maximum running speed because this pace couldn't be maintained for the entire distance. By now we hope you understand the differences between speed and power training.

Our second example is a also a combination power and speed workout for our willing subject, Lancetta, the female cyclist who is lucky to live in hill country. Her workout is shown in table 7.2. With cycling, as with running

TABLE 7.2 Sample Speed and Power Workout for a Cyclist*

Piece	Split time	Rest interval	Focus	Percent MHR
Warm-up	10 miles at 14 mph (16 km at 22 km/h)			<70% MHR
6 × 4:00 climbing	4:00	4:00–5:00 <60% MHR	Speed	95–100% MHR
Cool-down	10 miles (16 km)			<70% MHR

*Subject: 39-year-old female cyclist
MHR: 181 bpm
95–100% MHR = 172–181 bpm
<60% MHR = 109 bpm

and cross-country skiing, speed and power can be addressed in the same piece because of the climbing.

In this situation, Lancetta rides really hard and fast over very short distances at maximum effort and uses a full holiday to recover. During the rest interval, as she gets closer to fall-off-her-bike tired during each repeat, her heart rate takes longer to drop back down to 60 percent MHR, and so would look like this:

> 6 × 4 minutes in HR zone 172 to 181 bpm with an unspecified recovery time of very slow, easy peddling and coasting back down the hill to return her heart rate to less than 109 bpm

The nice thing about this approach is that it allows Lancetta to monitor her recovery objectively. As she takes longer to recover from the increasingly more difficult hill climbs, her heart rate will drop more slowly and the interval rest periods will get longer, another benefit of monitoring the right variable. Remember, asking an athlete to repeat speed or power workouts without adequate rest simply reduces the stimulus because the repeats get performed at lower speeds.

The main difference between the workout for the short-distance runner and Lancetta's workout is that one uses maximum power (40-meter and 75-meter sprints) to develop both speed and power, whereas the other uses high submaximum speed (but not maximum power), which will really target more speed than power. Again, if we go back and use the time parameters to guide our power-versus-speed session, you'll see that the cycling sessions

Edwin Moses: Early Heart Rate Pioneer

Here's another example of using a heart rate monitor to determine the givens and variables in training. This is a good real-life example of effort-based training. Edwin Moses, arguably the world's greatest all-time 400-meter hurdler, was an engineering student at Morehouse College in Atlanta. He took his interest in objectivity and numbers and adapted his workouts to heart rate measurements as well as anyone we've known.

During the fall season, Moses used his heart rate monitor to force him to do the kind of training that is the weakness of almost every sprinter: endurance and stamina training. Specifically, he worked on tempo runs for anaerobic threshold training on the Piedmont Park grass and hills. He performed cross-country-style, continuous workouts with his heart rate in his AT zone. During the track season in the spring and summer, he switched his monitoring to the recovery intervals between his speed work on the track. He never started speed or power repeats or sprints over the hurdles until his heart rate was fully recovered below 60 percent.

Moses lowered the world record several times, won two Olympic gold medals, and once had a streak of 122 straight victories in an event that is one of the hardest in track and field. You have to love those engineers and their heart rate monitors.

last several minutes versus several seconds. Both of these approaches are valuable in different ways. The decision of which one to use is often determined by how comfortable and safe it is for the person to move at maximum effort and velocity.

Smart athletes monitor what's going on. You need to be aware of the multiple methods available to improve your fitness and race performances. Coming up, we will look specifically at some techniques to improve speed and power.

Transition to Speed and Power Training

Before you go out and break the sound barrier, you must ask yourself this important question: Am I ready for interval or high-intensity training? For the most part, an athlete must be well conditioned before embarking on higher-intensity workouts. For runners, cross-country skiers, rowers, and other endurance athletes, a simple guideline is to time yourself for your best effort over about 5,000 meters. Pay attention to your 1,000-meter splits. If your last 1,000-meter split is about the same as your first 1,000-meter split, then you are probably ready for higher-intensity work. If it varies by more than 3 or 4 percent, you need further continuous, steady endurance work. Cyclists require a longer distance of about 10 miles (16 km) on a flat course applying the same logic (i.e., the first-mile split is similar to the last-mile split). For swimmers an appropriate distance would be 1 mile (1,600 meters) taking your first and last 200-meter splits.

Training Techniques to Develop Speed and Power

Transitioning into higher-intensity work is crucial for race performance. Several training approaches exist to help you accomplish your goals, including continuous distance work for aerobic base development, steady state and tempo training to transition into anaerobic work, and economy work to address race speed and anaerobic threshold changes. The acquisition of speed and power requires the elevation of AT and increased speed of movement. Speed training can take various forms:

- High-intensity, continuous exercise (often called pace running)
- Interval training with variable intensity efforts 80 to 175 percent max aerobic velocity (i.e., the maximum speed you can maintain for about three minutes)
- A combination of these two

Both interval training and high-intensity, continuous exercise require that you spend identified periods of time above your anaerobic threshold. To do this, you need a period of trial and error to determine the correct intensity (look back at Lancetta's economy and speed sessions for an example). Although heart rate is the best measure of intensity, it sometimes must be used concurrently with speed and pace.

At very high intensities, the ability to monitor and use heart rate as a guide becomes impaired because you elicit an MHR response across a range of intensities that exceed your maximum aerobic velocity. The heart rate response is also delayed because of the intense effort. Athletes, especially cyclists, runners, swimmers, and rowers, can easily use speed, in terms of minutes per mile/kilometer or miles/kilometers per hour, as a substitute measure. Many watches, computers, and GPS systems allow you to monitor speed in real time. For interval pieces and repeats that typically take place at or above race pace, you will quickly see that heart rate is maximal for many levels of the set pieces. As mentioned, HR response is delayed and does not yield sufficient information to allow you to determine intensity accurately. Therefore, for maximum pieces and near-maximum pieces (speed and power training), you should use both speed and heart rate to monitor intensity. Then you can also use heart rate to monitor your recovery interval and determine your readiness for the next piece.

You are probably familiar by now with the use of heart rate to monitor intensity. Using speed simply requires that you pay a little attention to the distances you are covering and the time in which you are covering them. You can do this by using timing splits. For example, let's say you are a cross-country skier with a goal time of less than 21 minutes for a certain 5K course

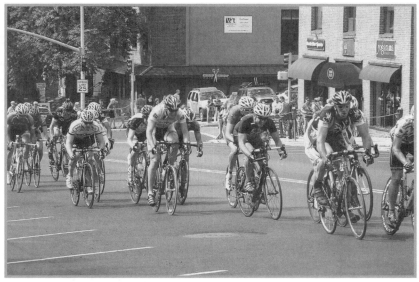

Declan Connolly

Cyclists can measure speed or watts (power) instead of heart rate during intense efforts that negatively affect the ability to take accurate readings with a heart rate monitor.

that is fairly flat (cross-country ski courses vary dramatically with terrain).

We break this into five 1-kilometer segments. You must average 4:12 per kilometer. Using this target of 4:12, you can perform 1-kilometer pieces at or below this target to allow you to move at the required speed. This would be an example of using speed rather than heart rate to guide intensity. You could then use heart rate to guide your recovery.

High-Intensity, Continuous Exercise

The first approach to developing speed is high-intensity, continuous exercise (HICE). These workouts are similar to tempo exercises. However, instead of keeping the effort and heart rate constant while slowing down the pace over the latter parts of the tempo workout, HICE workouts keep the pace the same and push the heart rate higher until it reaches maximum. In short, HICE workouts are like time trials or even races.

A HICE workout requires that you perform 20 minutes or more, depending on your sport, at an intensity level well above AT—for example, starting with intensities at 90 to 95 percent MHR and ending close to 100 percent MHR. How long the exercise session lasts varies greatly from sport to sport and will also determine the intensity level. Cyclists appear to be able to perform at maximum levels for longer periods of times than runners can, whereas rowers and swimmers are behind runners. We're not entirely sure why this is, but it may have something to do with the more complex skills required in the latter sports. The intensity level should allow you to complete the exercise session just before fatigue or exhaustion sets in. Thus, HICE workouts usually use distances that are shorter than race distances because the intensity is higher.

HICE is designed to simulate racing conditions in terms of tempo and effort except that the speed is faster. This can be done because the distance covered is shorter. HICE also allows you to work on form and mechanics as you try to maintain form while fatigue sets in. A mistake athletes often make is to have HICE sessions that are too fast and therefore too short.

In deciding the intensity and duration of HICE pieces, we like to use the one-third, one-third, one-third mentality. The first third should be relatively comfortable, to the point that you may say to yourself, "I could actually run much faster." During the second third, you should start thinking about getting tired and maintaining your form, but you are still okay in terms of pain. In the final third, you are just hanging in there and trying not to have everything fall apart. Selecting your pace is crucial because a pace elicits very different responses toward the end of the run than it did at the beginning. One HICE session a week is enough for the average person.

Here is an example of a HICE session. Let's say a runner has a goal of running a 10K in 50 minutes (about 8:04 per mile). It is reasonable to assume that he can run a 5K in 25 minutes. However, because a 5K is much shorter, this actually represents a lower overall intensity. If this runner were to perform a HICE session over 5K, he might instead select a goal time of 23:45

The Great Lactate Debate

Perhaps no other area in sport performance and training has received as much negative publicity as lactic acid. Lactic acid is blamed for fatigue, exhaustion, muscle soreness, muscle damage, overtraining, and more. But is it really all that bad? Is it even worth this much attention?

Blood lactate profiling is commonly used by upper-level coaches and athletes to monitor training quality and quantity. Lactate measurement requires knowledge of the athlete's lactate threshold (LT), commonly defined as the intensity of exercise above which lactic acid noticeably accumulates. Why would this be important to know? Theoretically, if the lactate concentration is accumulating, then the athlete is on borrowed time because the concentration will eventually be high enough to compromise energy production and muscle action. This theory relies on the belief that lactate concentration actually does limit both energy production and muscle action.

Athletes vary immensely in their peak lactate concentrations depending on their training state, muscle fiber composition, and even diet. Some athletes generate peak lactate values of 16 to 17 mmol/L, whereas some generate peak levels of 11 to 12 mmol/L. Clearly, there is high interindividual variation in this response. If lactate monitoring is to be used at all, individual profiles must be developed independent of standardized guidelines. Unfortunately, the 4 mmol/L mark is widely and generically referred to as the LT regardless of individual variation or measurement. Furthermore, resting lactate values vary in athletes from 0.9 mmol/L to 2.9 mmol/L, leaving a wide difference in the amount of lactate response among individuals to get to the 4mmol/L. Lactate data are even less accurate in athletes younger than 17 years old.

Lactate measurement has become relatively easy and inexpensive. However, it still requires scientific precision and accuracy. A lack of precision and accuracy is a major downfall for most coaches. Lack of control over blood volumes, sweat contamination, air exposure time, and athlete rest contribute to inconsistency and inaccuracy. Initial profiling is best done under laboratory conditions where most of these variables can be controlled.

So is it worthwhile to monitor lactate? Yes and no. Yes, if you are sure you're getting good data, but no, if you're not. The majority of lactate data we collect in athletes younger than 16 is inconsistent and tells us little. Also, how much does lactate explain?

At the University of Vermont we completed a study that looked at power production over consecutive bouts under two conditions: active and passive recovery. We also monitored lactate over six consecutive bouts. Active recovery yielded greater power output, but lactate was not different between the conditions, suggesting that high concentrations of lactate alone could not explain fatigue. What implications does this have for training?

Some scientists assert that velocity at LT is the most accurate predictor of performance. If so, two scenarios are possible. First, a person with a low peak lactate concentration may be able to move faster before LT occurs at the 4 mmol/L mark. Second, a person with a high peak lactate concentration may be able to move faster at LT because he can sustain higher LTs. It seems contradictory. However, the contradiction lies in the belief that LT is 4 mmol/L for all athletes. This likely is not true. Rather, it varies among athletes and needs to be scientifically determined using additional physiological markers such as ventilation and volume of carbon dioxide production. Combining these factors to determine true LT is necessary before you can rely on lactate measurement. Even then, it is unwise to rely on it as your sole source of monitoring intensity.

(continued)

for the 5K, thereby reducing the mile splits to 7:38 per mile, or about 1:54 per quarter mile.

The ending heart rate would be the same for both the 10K and the 5K— maximal, but reached after 23:45 instead of 50:00. If you understand this logic, you can put together a HICE session for any length you want.

Here's a second example of a subject who wants to run a half marathon in less than 2:10:00. This puts the mile splits at about 9:55 per mile. A HICE session might be 7 miles at 9:30 per mile or even 9:15 per mile. Again, maximum heart rate would be achieved at the end of both the half marathon and the 7 miles.

Here's an example of a rower. Let's say a rower sets a goal of 40 minutes for a 10K piece. Rowers commonly use 500-meter split times, so this would equate to a 2-minute split per 500 meters. This means a rower could easily row 5K in 20 minutes, but setting a HICE goal might reduce the 500-meter split to 1:52, giving the rower a 5K time of 18:40. Again, in both cases the session demands a maximum effort with the same ending MHR, but under two different conditions.

So we can see that HICE is a good way to introduce speed and high-intensity work. However, it doesn't really work for power; for that we turn to intervals.

Interval Training

With interval training, you spend varying periods of time above AT but usually at a much higher intensity overall. In fact, interval speed is always significantly higher than race pace because it is for a shorter duration. This is much like HICE training, except intervals usually are done at higher speeds and, more important, include a recovery.

Look back at the speed and power table for the 5K runner (table 7.1, page 90) for an example of an interval training session. Intervals are different from HICE in that they are not continuous; instead, they involve a series of work pieces split by recovery intervals. The ratio of work to rest is variable and can be adjusted accordingly to allow a greater or lesser number of work pieces in a session. Again, look back at the scenarios of Lancetta and Edwin Moses for examples of using heart rate as the recovery guideline. In these scenarios we used 60 percent of MHR as the target for when the athlete was recovered. Often coaches use both time and heart rate for a recovery guideline as the heart rate becomes the minimum standard for heart-rate recovery while the time can be used to ensure recovery. For example, a coach might use recovery heart rate less that 60 percent MHR plus 30 seconds as the entire recovery interval.

Intervals do not need to be of the same length or intensity within an exercise session but should probably be designed with shorter distances in the middle or at the end of the session. Intervals are also of value because they train you to move fast. Some may argue that this can compromise technique if not controlled. However, you should be able to focus on good technique because the periods are shorter. Furthermore, if your technique is compromised, then your coach will have identified an additional concern—that you cannot maintain good form at higher work rates. (Swimmers have successfully trained this way for many years.) Varying-length intervals are more productive because they help you gauge effort, pacing, and strategy, while also helping you focus mentally in different situations.

Remember, intervals requiring you to perform faster than race pace must be strategically scheduled. This increased speed is central to the interval approach, and because the time spent at speeds faster than race pace is less than the time of an actual race, you can probably handle it (again, see Lancetta's strategy).

Table 7.3 shows laboratory data collected from a runner. The example that follows shows how we would use the physiological data collected to design an appropriate high-intensity session.

TABLE 7.3 Physiological Data for a Male Runner

Age	41
Mass	71 kg
Height	170 cm
MHR predicted (220 – age)	179 bpm
True MHR	182 bpm
% max AT	80%
$\dot{V}O_2$max	58 ml/kg/min^{-1}
HR at AT	163 bpm
$\dot{V}O_2$ at AT	47 ml/kg/min^{-1}
400 m split max	58 sec
Mile pace at AT	7:45 min
5K best	20:46 min

This athlete's AT occurs at a heart rate of about 163 bpm, or at a 7:45 mile pace. (A simple guideline for AT if you cannot scientifically measure it is to do the talk test. When conversing is problematic, or you go quiet, you're around AT.) We can use these numbers to create threshold workouts. As the heart rate selected for the work rate increases, the time for the work piece normally decreases. Alternatively, the runner could run at less than 163 bpm per mile for more than 60 minutes. Regardless, we know for this athlete that effective speed and threshold work must occur at greater than 163 bpm and at a split less than 7:45 per mile.

With HICE, the heart rate will creep up slowly over the duration of the workout even though the speed is the same. This phenomenon is called *cardiovascular drift* or *cardiovascular creep* and in most cases is a function of increasing body temperature. It can be offset with regular fluid replenishment (this was discussed in chapter 4). Therefore, workout intensity may have to be adjusted to compensate for cardiovascular drift, and this is easily done by slightly decreasing intensity. For continuous exercise sessions of shorter duration, the intensity must be correspondingly increased. For example, if the session is only 20 minutes, then the sample athlete might elect to start at a heart rate of 170 bpm or more. Remember, in HICE sessions the athlete should approach maximum effort at the end of the session. The bottom line: They are very difficult workouts!

When to Start Interval Training or HICE

Interval and HICE workouts require a solid aerobic foundation, which normally requires 12 to 16 weeks of training. Typically, a solid aerobic foundation is developed in the off-season or winter season. Because higher-intensity training is more demanding, it necessitates a decrease in volume and is not unlike a tapering program. In fact, many successful athletes use intervals as part of their tapering programs, and numerous scientific studies have documented the effectiveness of tapering programs that use only high-intensity, low-volume training. Therefore, high-intensity sessions should begin in earnest about 8 to 10 weeks prior to competition. The success of these sessions also requires a degree of metabolic enzyme adaptation, and this takes less time than the basic musculoskeletal adaptation to the increased intensity. A goal of intervals or HICE is to begin a simulation of race intensity and mental state. If we put the previous scenario into a 24-week training program, it would look something like this:

- 16 weeks of lower-intensity steady-state work five days a week to build the aerobic base
- 4 weeks of four steady-state days and one HICE day
- 4 weeks of three steady-state days, one HICE day, and one interval day

Workout Pattern for Speed and Power Development

When starting higher-intensity training, you should schedule only one session per week for about three to four weeks. This will allow adaptation to the new speed. Then schedule two sessions each week at least three days apart. Generally, two of these sessions a week are enough at any level, and progression can come in the form of either a shorter interval rest period or a faster piece.

When you put your program together, you'll find that there are often more types of workouts than days of the week to fit them in. As a general rule, we suggest that when you reach a satisfactory fitness level based on five days a week, you should devote three days to steady endurance work and two days to speed. This might result in one interval day and one HICE day out of a five-day training week. Older athletes will definitely find more than two high-intensity sessions a week hard to recover from.

Recovery Between High-Intensity Workouts

The question often arises about how much recuperation time is required between training sessions. Naturally, this depends on the intensity of the session, whether you performed more than one session in one day, your age, and perhaps most important, your dietary practices. Arguably, the most important time to eat is immediately following exercise, especially after high-intensity exercise that is primarily carbohydrate dependent. The quality of this food intake is of paramount importance in determining the degree of carbohydrate repletion in the muscle. A general guideline is that carbohydrate replenishment takes at least 24 hours. Therefore, consecutive days of hard intervals are not advised; usually two days between sessions (such as a Monday and Thursday schedule) allows for adequate recovery. Older athletes need to be even more conservative about scheduling intervals because recovery will take a little longer. Table 7.4 shows a simple schematic of how a weekly program might look at this phase of training.

The program outlined in table 7.4 allows you to mix up speed, power, and endurance sessions. It also allows you to target both maximum speed and submaximum speed by doing a day of HICE and then another of intervals. Performing two days a week of endurance will allow you to preserve that hard-earned endurance base with a slightly faster economy run also included to remind you of race pace. A well-balanced session like this will also provide adequate recovery days so you can put in a fair effort during all exercise sessions. You will notice that we have inserted recovery days following both speed workouts because these typically require a little longer recovery.

The bottom line with race training is that you need to run fast to run faster. Rowing fast, running fast, biking fast, swimming fast, and so on, require

TABLE 7.4 Sample Weekly Program That Incorporates High-Intensity Workouts		
Day	**Focus**	**Method**
Monday	Speed	HICE
Tuesday	Off	
Wednesday	Endurance	LSD
Thursday	Speed	Interval
Friday	Off	
Saturday	Economy	Tempo
Sunday	Endurance	LSD

physiological, psychological, and biomechanical effort. Such effort is also uncomfortable, and for many athletes, this can be the greatest challenge. At higher work intensities the breathing discomfort, the heaviness in the legs and arms, and the burning in the chest are real. These are race-like symptoms. Spending time moving fast, above AT and approaching maximum heart and breathing rates, while also enduring the effort, will help prepare you for the race environment. When you have accomplished all of the base and foundation work, the next step is higher-intensity work, and there isn't really any way to prepare for competition than to perform a combination of high-intensity workouts. However, you should plan properly and base your sessions on your own unique data.

As a final note, think about and plan the recovery time for your intervals very carefully. The recovery times are arguably more important than the work times because they regulate the quality of your work output. If you get too little rest, fatigue comes quickly; if you get too much rest, the stimulus for change is reduced. Anyone can make an athlete tired, but not everyone can make that athlete faster.

PART III

PROGRAMS

CHAPTER 8

Designing an Effective Training Program

By this stage, we have covered most of the background information you need to use your heart rate monitor accurately. In part III of the book, we present examples of training programs for a number of sports. At this point we need to consider the elements of a program and the factors to consider when designing one.

Your training program will serve as your daily guideline and as such will have to be organized weeks and months in advance. You have many factors to consider, ranging from the more straightforward elements of frequency, time, and duration (which we'll cover shortly) to the more complex aspects of energy systems and making sure they are all appropriately developed to allow maximum performance. You will recall from chapter 1 the training triangle that depicts a solid aerobic, or endurance, base to be developed before anything else; developing that base also takes up the most amount of time. All programs start with building the solid base, which comprises lots of low intensity or easy volume. From there the building continues into the higher-intensity threshold work and finally into the red zone where intensity is very high and speed is very fast.

You also remember the four training phases that specifically target endurance, stamina, economy, and speed. These phases span the spectrum of energy systems ranging from very aerobic to slightly anaerobic (economy) to highly anaerobic (power). The training triangle emphasizes the importance of developing your systems progressively; you can develop your anaerobic systems only after you have developed an appropriate endurance (aerobic) base.

Depending on your initial level of fitness, developing an adequate aerobic base can take anywhere from 4 to 20 weeks. As a general rule, we classify aerobic fitness according to maximum oxygen consumption values. This data is presented in chapter 10 (page 125). However, because most of us do not have access to the technology required to measure such values, we provided a classification table (table 8.1) that uses a more accessible method of time for a 5K. Using this table, you can figure out whether you are a beginner (needing 16 to 20 weeks), at the intermediate level (needing 12 to 16 weeks), or advanced (needing 4 to 12 weeks).

Now that you have a sense of how to organize programs, it is time to look at some of the other factors and terms related to program design.

TABLE 8.1 5K Race Times for Runners at Different Levels	
Beginner	>29:30
Novice	22:30–29:29
Advanced	<22:29

Factors in Program Design

As we move on in our discussion of training and using heart rate, we want to make sure you understand some of the related training concepts and variables you must consider when developing a training program. Heart rate, although an extremely important variable, is only one measuring tool. To design a good program, you should also understand the following eight basic, straightforward principles of exercise prescription:

1. Frequency
2. Intensity
3. Duration
4. Mode
5. Overload
6. Specificity
7. Reversibility
8. Maintenance

Collectively, these eight principles dictate your current level of fitness. Let's look at each principle in more detail.

Frequency is simply a measure of how many times you exercise in a week. Basic fitness guidelines advise three to five times per week. However, this can vary significantly depending on the interaction between intensity and duration. As a general rule, beginners should exercise three or four times per week with a rest day scheduled every other day. Intermediate athletes should exercise four to seven times a week. Advanced athletes may exercise up to 15 times a week. More competitive athletes often exercise twice a day, incorporating one aerobic session and one weightlifting session, for example—or one session may be slow and the other fast. The bottom line is that virtually all of the more competitive athletes exercise more than seven times a week.

Intensity is simply a measure of how hard you work. However, your intensity must be planned and correlated with your progression. In chapter 1, we showed that intensity can be measured by percent MHR (maximum heart rate) or percent $\dot{V}O_2$max. Heart rate is the simplest and most effective tool for guiding intensity. You can ensure the adaptation you need for the training phase you are in by selecting the appropriate intensity. People often exercise too hard too early in their training programs and then get injured or fail to develop the appropriate foundation needed for higher intensity later on. Classifying yourself properly from the beginning will guide you in selecting the right intensity.

Duration is simply the length of the exercise session, the interval, or the piece. As a general rule, the longer the duration, the greater the intensity. Duration becomes an intensity factor over time. Even if you do something at low intensity, if you do it long enough, it becomes harder. Duration is important because it is very often manipulated to ensure a certain intensity stimulus. It also determines whether you will need to refuel your energy during an exercise session. Duration and intensity are closely intertwined.

Mode simply refers to the type of activity you do. Running, swimming, and biking are all examples of exercise modes. Mode is relevant for the development of efficiency, especially mechanical and metabolic efficiency. It also has implications for energy expended because different activities burn calories at different rates, even if the heart rate is the same. We also can be at different intensities or perceived efforts in different modes while exhibiting the same heart rate. Triathletes often notice greater comfort running at a heart rate of 140 bpm versus biking or swimming at 140 bpm.

The four factors discussed so far—frequency, intensity, duration, and mode—are the four core principles that are essential in the initial design of any exercise program. The next four components are more concerned with the progression of the program.

Overload refers to the increased demand placed on the muscular system. It simply means requiring the system to do more. Overload, sometimes referred to as progression, is also concerned with how much you increase your volume or intensity. As a general rule, novice and intermediate athletes should not increase volume by more than 10 percent in any given session during a two- to three-week period. This increase also assumes a minimum of three exercise sessions each week. In other words, you should do at least eight exercise sessions in a row at the same load before implementing any increases.

For example, let's say a beginner runs Monday, Wednesday, and Friday. She runs 3 miles (4.8 km) a day for a total of 9 (14.5 km) miles a week. After two weeks, this mileage would increase to approximately 10.5 miles (17 km) a week, or three runs at 3.5 miles (5.6 km) each. This progression model is slow, but it helps prevent injury and muscle damage while also allowing adequate time for multiple systems to adapt to the new overload. Using percentage of volume to increase overload is difficult because of the small amounts of increase. Instead, you can use time, which is easier to measure and monitor.

Specificity has two considerations—metabolic specificity and muscle contraction specificity. Specificity is concerned with putting the correct type of stress on your metabolic and musculoskeletal systems. For example, have you ever seen a really good runner struggle to swim 400 meters in the pool? Essentially, we become efficient at specific muscle contractions through practice and training. For runners this might require sprint work, for cyclists it might be hill work, and for triathletes it might involve working on transitions. The bottom line is that specificity has to do with coordinating your central nervous system to work in conjunction with your metabolic demands during muscular contractions. For many athletes this requires training at various speeds and intensities and in the mode that is most important. Of particular importance in this category is speed work, but again, only when the endurance base has been built.

Reversibility relates to losing whatever fitness you gained. The time course for losing fitness varies among athletes and types of fitness. For example, aerobic fitness begins to decline without any exercise in about 10 days. Muscular strength will not decline for about 30 days. Athletes often have a hard time grasping this concept because they believe that within one or two days the system starts to reverse and fitness is lost. Consequently, many athletes do not rest appropriately for important races, especially long races such as marathons or Ironman. The bottom line is that well-trained aerobic athletes do not lose any fitness for at least seven days. In fact, with appropriate rest, they will even improve performance, which is what we refer to as tapering. Remember, the hard part is getting fit; staying fit is a bit easier.

Maintenance and reversibility are somewhat linked. Maintenance simply refers to the maintenance of your current fitness. Maintenance of fitness is achieved with much less work and effort than improving fitness. Maintenance of fitness can actually be achieved with a 30 to 40 percent decrease in volume provided you are happy with not getting any better or any faster. During the tapering phases of training, you can actually decrease your volume up to 80 percent provided that you keep the intensity very high (usually greater than 90 percent of MHR). This is why many athletes dramatically cut volume but increase speed and intensity in the weeks leading up to big races, yet still race faster.

Now that you understand these programming principles, let's consider how you can manipulate them during training using heart rate training zones. Remember, you are trying to build a logical and systematic program to develop the elements of power, speed, and endurance that you need—and do it without getting hurt.

Periodization

Before we get into the real nuts and bolts of building the program, we want to take a look at the big picture of a training program. We refer to this as periodization, and it describes the organization of an overall training program. The program might be 12 weeks long, 6 months long, or 1 year long. For Olympic athletes, it might be 4 years long. Regardless of the length of time, the program is organized around the scientific principles of progression. If you plan your periodization correctly, you will find that you can align heart rate intensities with periods in the cycle for the most part. The longer, slower, base-building cycles will be characterized by much lower heart rates overall and essentially display the phase I endurance zones. As you move into higher-intensity cycles, your heart rate will elevate.

A well-organized program focuses on different components of overall fitness during different periods—macrocycles, microcycles, and mesocycles. The four phases of training—endurance, stamina, economy, and speed—fit within these periods. In general, macrocycles are longer, or more generally defined, periods of training that lack the specificity and detail of microcycles and mesocycles. For example, a macrocycle in a six-month training program might comprise the first 12 weeks of simple, low-intensity aerobic conditioning designed to build an endurance base.

Microcycles are shorter periods with an increased focus on another aspect of fitness. For example, in a six-month training program in which the first 12 weeks are a macrocycle, two microcycles of four weeks each might follow. These microcycles might include a focus on speed work, hill work, tempo runs, or flexibility. During microcycles we tend to focus a little more on the specific components required for performance and racing.

Mesocycles are the final part of the periodization process. These are individual sessions designed to address a particular skill component. A mesocycle for a runner might focus on pacing, tempo running, or mechanics. For a cyclist, a mesocycle might focus on body position or climbing posture. For a swimmer, it might focus on stroke technique.

The use of periodization forces you to consider in detail the type of adaptations you are looking for during a particular phase of your program. It forces you to be organized, consider how long you have to adapt, and decide where the competition occurs in your overall training program. When designing an exercise program, you should be looking at the desired end point, or product. Ask yourself, "What am I looking for in terms of performance at the end of the training program?" When you can define that, you can work backward to ensure that the correct amount of time is available to ensure the adaptations needed. This prevents you from making the basic mistake of progressing too rapidly and increasing your risk of injury.

If you look back at the general structure of a training program through the lens of periodization, you will see that more general conditioning sessions occur early on (macrocycles), and that these become progressively more specific (microcycles and mesocycles). Within each of these periods you will also see variations in intensity, distance, recovery, and so on. Here again, heart rate is your guiding tool to ensure that you stay within the parameters of intensity you need to get the appropriate adaptation. Clearly, being organized and plotting out your program is paramount.

Principle of Progressive Resistance

The principle of progressive resistance can be applied to either slow or fleet-footed movements. This primary law of physiology states that we can condition our muscles by working them with repetitive movements to a state of fatigue and then overloading them with a few more repetitions.

The most familiar application of this principle is weight training. We all know that lifting weights can make you stronger. Perhaps you are familiar with the two ways to weight train: lift a light weight many times or lift a heavy weight a few times. Either one works, but only if the weight is lifted enough times or is heavy enough for 100 percent of the muscle fibers to be recruited into action, almost reach failure, and then be made to overload to the quiver, struggle, and burn level.

Although there are important secondary fitness benefits to both of the weight training choices, let's consider a standard set of 10 repetitions (or reps) as an example. A set of 10 reps is both safe and efficient for improving strength. Start by selecting, through trial and error, the amount of weight that will fatigue your muscle group within seven reps. The overload that occurs with the eighth, ninth, and tenth reps stimulates adaptation. Once the muscle is strong enough to move that weight 10 times without reaching overload, increase the resistance to reach the next level of fitness and strength. How long this process continues depends on your goal, but more resistance in the form of heavier weights is necessary to get stronger. For example, if Larry Lifter found that he could reach overload with 95 pounds (43 kg) when doing bench presses, once he could do his set of 10 reps, he would next add 10 pounds (4.5 kg) to reach the new overload. This process would continue to 115 pounds (52 kg) once he could not overload with 105 pounds (48 kg).

Now, let's apply the principles of progressive resistance training to walking, jogging, and running. In fact, you can extend this example creatively to any of the endurance sports. The resistance for these activities is the body's weight against gravity. However, you won't be moving heavier weights to increase the resistance. In fact, as you get in better shape, you may actually move less weight. Therefore, you have three choices to increase resistance:

1. Lengthen the duration of the exercise sessions—walk, jog, or run farther at the same pace.

2. Add more intensity by lifting your weight higher against gravity—walk, jog, or run faster.

3. Add more intensity by changing the degree of incline—head for the hills.

In other words, getting stronger and fitter by walking is like a lifting a very light weight many times. Jogging is like lifting the next increment of still fairly light weights not quite so many times. Running is like lifting heavy weights fewer times. Running up hills is like lifting the maximum weight just a few times.

Workouts at slower paces in lower-intensity heart rate zones will take more time, whereas faster workouts in higher-intensity zones will be over more quickly. Your heart rate, patience, and goals will determine how much or how little time you spend.

Monitoring Progress and Recovery

By now the concept of monitoring heart rate is familiar to you. You also know that increased duration represents increased intensity and that, generally, increases in duration lead to poor recovery. However, because we know that heart rate is extremely versatile and responsive, we can use it to monitor both acute and chronic recovery as well as adaptations. In the next section we take a look at both acute and chronic heart rate responses and consider how they can be used to regulate intensity and recovery within an exercise session and also guide recovery between workouts to prevent overtraining.

Using Acute Heart Rate to Guide Recovery Within an Exercise Session

Heart rate response during exercise is typically a reflection of the intensity of the exercise. During an exercise session, you may experience several increases in intensity that cause a higher heart rate, such as after you climb a hill. It also happens during speed interval sessions on the track. You may have to slow down or stop after this brief period of increased intensity to recover to some degree. An important question at this point is: When are you ready to perform the next interval? Your within-exercise recovery heart rate is the answer.

You can determine when you are ready to start up again by monitoring your recovery heart rate. As a general rule, 65 percent MHR is used as the criterion for adequate recovery. However, this is not a hard-and-fast rule. If you are doing high-intensity speed or power workouts that last only a few seconds, your coach might select a 50 percent recovery rate for 800-meter intervals. The bottom line with recovery heart rates is that you must achieve enough recovery to allow you to perform your complete workout with sufficient quality rather than at significantly reduced speeds or efforts. Generally, fitter athletes use higher percentages of MHR while recovering.

Your appropriate heart rate recovery depends on how much and how well you want to recover between bouts. In general, the faster or the higher the intensity of the exercise piece, the greater your recovery should be. So, for example, if you are running intervals at 85 percent MHR, you would need less recovery than if you were running intervals at 95 to 100 percent MHR.

Here's an example. A coach might select a 50 percent MHR target as a recovery number. When the athlete's heart rate drops back down to that level, she can resume the workload or perform the next piece. Here is an easy math example: A 20-year-old runner has a maximum heart rate of 200 bpm. The session comprises ten 200-meter repeats on the track. Following the repeats, the coach can use time or heart rate to determine when the athlete should start up again. Some coaches use a combination of both. In the current example, the coach does not have the athlete perform the next 200 meters until her heart rate drops below 100 bpm (50 percent of the maximum heart rate). This is an example of using acute heart rate response during recovery when monitoring heart rate solely within a given exercise session.

Using Chronic Heart Rate to Guide Recovery Within an Exercise Session

Changes in heart rate measurement technology now allow us to collect data for much longer periods extending beyond the exercise session (over 24 hours at a time). Because we can monitor heart rate over longer periods, we can get excellent resting and recovery data between days of exercise. (You could refer to this as daily heart rate recovery.) This can guide daily training intensities and allow you to make changes if you're not fully recovered from the previous exercise bout.

Look back at figure 1.2 (page 10) to see this depicted. Here is an example to illustrate this point. Let's say you get into the habit of recording resting heart rate, and your average heart rate when you wake up in the morning is 52 bpm. On Sunday you do a 10-mile (16 km) run. You wake up on Monday with a resting heart rate of 55 bpm. You choose to go ahead with a scheduled track and speed session (low volume but high intensity) on Monday. When you wake up Tuesday morning, your resting heart rate is 56 bpm. This is an indication that you have not recovered from the Sunday workout (and Monday added to the dilemma) and that you should implement either a very easy workout on Tuesday or take a complete rest day. This is why good record keeping is useful. Using this approach, within one to two days your resting heart rate should recover. If it does not, you may have a more serious problem of overtraining or staleness on your hands. This will necessitate longer periods of rest and strategic nutrition.

If you pay close attention to your heart rate not only during exercise but also on a daily basis, you will get a lot of feedback about your overall state of recovery and readiness for the next training session. This will also help reduce the likelihood of injury.

Avoiding Overtraining and Staleness

Overtraining and staleness can be avoided by monitoring heart rate. Bear in mind that overtraining is a complex area. However, you can use heart rate data to indicate too much training in the early stages, what we refer to as acute overtraining, or overreaching.

Overreaching applies to short-term overtraining, as might happen after a particularly hard training session. This usually occurs in the few days following a longer, more strenuous workout. Overtraining applies to longer, more chronic overtraining conditions that result after weeks or months of training without adequate rest and nutrition. This is a more serious condition requiring lengthy periods of rest, nutrition, and perhaps medical intervention. In contrast, overreaching can normally be addressed with a few days of rest and a few hearty meals.

Using your heart rate monitor can keep you from developing either overtraining condition. To use it effectively, you need to do two things:

1. Record and monitor your resting heart rate and exercise heart rate response to a given workload as often as possible. These should be documented over days, weeks, and months.

2. Understand how your heart rate should respond both at rest and during exercise as you train. Make sure it is increasing and decreasing as you would expect.

Addressing the first issue is fairly straightforward. The second requires that you read on a little further. Under normal conditions, resting heart rate should be back to normal within 24 hours of a workout. You should make sure this is the case before proceeding with a higher-intensity workload the following day. Over time, however, your heart rate should decrease both at rest and in response to a fixed workload. The decreased heart rate response under both situations is a result of improved cardiac muscle function—the heart is stronger and can move more blood with each beat. We call this increased stroke volume. If you are not fully recovered, then your heart rate at rest will be elevated because it is still working at repairing tissues and replenishing fuels. What's more, if you are not recovered, your heart rate during exercise will not increase to where it needs to be to supply the needed blood flow. This results in the sluggishness or staleness athletes often experience during early overreaching. It feels as though someone has put the lid on the heart rate. As a result, you try to work harder but cannot because the heart rate cannot elevate to give you the blood supply you need. The result is a frustrating and psychologically damaging workout. Your legs and arms are heavy, and the best thing you can do is go home, eat, and sleep.

It is nice to have your 12-week program carved in stone. However, you need to be open-minded enough to change your daily plan if your body needs it. The question is, What should you do if your heart rate indicates overtraining? The obvious answer to is simply to cut back on the volume of exercise you are doing, especially for the next few days. For some athletes this is not always possible, but there are a few other precautions you can take.

The first step is to determine whether you are in an acute stage of overtraining or overreaching, or whether these are early symptoms of a more long-term, chronic problem. To determine this, we ask athletes three questions. (1) Are you finding your exercise sessions getting more difficult or easier? If they are getting more difficult and they are the same workouts (i.e., same speed), you're overtraining. (2) Are you very tired but having trouble getting good-quality sleep? If so, you are overtraining. (3) Do you find it difficult to exert maximum effort during a routine training session? If so, you're overtraining. These three simple questions will help you determine whether you are starting to overtrain.

Early stages of overtraining are really overreaching. Overreaching generally occurs when there is a marked increase in intensity or volume, which quite often happens to athletes attending training camp where there is a significant increase in workload within a short period of time. The good news about overreaching is that it can be addressed relatively quickly and easily, with three or four days of planned rest and appropriate nutritional intervention.

Ignoring the symptoms and continuing to train with the mentality that you just need to grind through the sessions will inevitably lead to classic overtraining. Classic overtraining is a more long-term problem with more serious consequences. It usually has all the signs and symptoms of overreaching plus a couple more: resting heart rate continues to be elevated at rest, and exercise heart rates continue to be depressed despite efforts to work harder. What follows tends to be a period of illness or sickness as a result of a compromised immune system. At this point you are clearly overtraining and facing several weeks or possibly several months of layoff from exercise.

Fortunately, by monitoring your heart rate regularly both at rest and during exercise, you can detect these early symptoms. Then, you can take appropriate action to vary the intensity and duration of workouts to ensure that you do not move from the overreaching condition into the overtraining condition.

One of the keys to ensuring that you do not overtrain is to consider your abilities, nutrition, age, and recovery profiles when designing your training program. An individually designed program will enable you to detect early whether you are overreaching and overtraining. Developing appropriate training programs requires an understanding of progression, duration, intensity, and the other factors. You also need to clearly identify the length of the training program. From there the program should be built using the foundations described in chapter 1.

Putting It Together

We have covered the elements to consider in program design. Now we can think about piecing together this puzzle. Look at the flowchart in figure 8.1 for an overall picture of what the program might look like in terms of time focused on particular fitness components. We find it is helpful to plot out your time frames generically and then go back into those sections and add greater detail. Doing so results in a more detailed training program such as the example provided for the 1,500-meter runner (table 8.2). Workouts designed to address specific components are detailed in the microcycle piece.

To design an effective program, you need to know the type of adaptations that must occur during the various cycles of the program. In general, we recognize several cycles that must occur in an overall training program: the base cycle (the endurance-building cycle); a competition cycle; and a recovery, or transition, cycle. A program that clearly defines each of these phases will result in sound progression. It will allow you to peak at the right time. It will also ensure that you have an appropriate taper phase. As you look at the

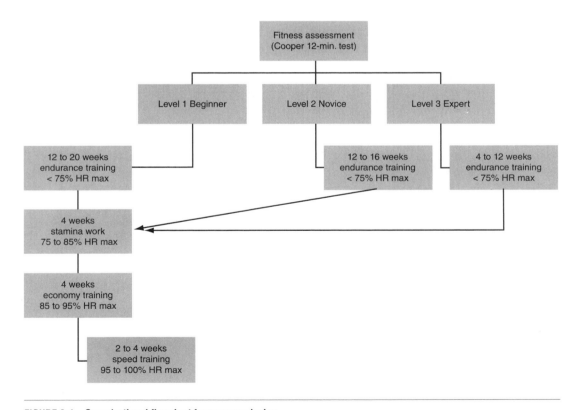

FIGURE 8.1 **Organizational flowchart for program design.**

TABLE 8.2 Year-Long Periodization Plan for a 1,500-Meter Runner

Sub-phases	Phases					
	Preparation endurance and stamina (12-16 weeks)		Competition speed (4 weeks)		Recuperation (4-8 weeks)	Early transition (12-20 weeks)
Macro-cycle	Volume endur-ance	Intensity stamina	Speed HICE economy	Power sprints speed	Fun/cross-train Active rest	Aerobic/skill development Low intensity/high volume Endurance
Micro-cycle						

programs for the various sports, remember that the same logic and organization applies for all sports. Always start with the low-intensity endurance, or base-building, phase, which is the longest phase. Then, methodically and patiently move through the more specific, higher-intensity phases, which are shorter. The general model is the same for all sports. The only variations are those that need to occur because of specific movement patterns required by the sport. For example, in swimming, more time might be spent doing drills.

CHAPTER 9

Walking

The previous chapters delivered a great deal of theory as well as practical advice on monitored training and its application to exercising in general. The submaximum nature of walking, the activity covered in this chapter, requires some exceptions to the concepts discussed previously. Creative alternatives are needed. For example, although you will use percentage of maximum heart rate (MHR) to determine your training zones, you will use a special, perhaps slightly less than fully maximum heart rate. The challenge is to find a lower zone of intensity that will still accomplish the goals of improving endurance and stamina.

Your training zones will have wide ranges. You may need to rely on your own perception of your effort to verify that the heart rates you see are, indeed, reliable and effective. You'll still use your heart rate to determine how far, how fast, and how hard you should work out. This approach should be both easy to follow and challenging.

In this chapter, you will learn to apply the overload principle of progressive resistance to your walking. Just as someone must lift a light weight many times to get stronger, walkers must take a lot of steps to reach the point of muscle overload because of the rather weak challenge to gravity. By comparison, sprinting is like lifting a heavy weight a few times to reach muscle overload. In either case, you can track the oxygen demands of your working muscles by keeping track of your cardiac system's response in heartbeats per minute.

Have you been enjoying enough casual, unstructured walking long enough to be able to comfortably walk at least 20 minutes two or three times a week and take one longer stroll of 30 minutes once a week? Furthermore, during one of your 20-minute walks, can you cover at least 1 mile (1.6 km)? If so, then read on. This program is not designed for rank beginners who are just sliding off the couch. If you don't meet the prerequisite of 20 minutes two or three times a week (one of them for at least 1 mile, or 1.6 km) and a 30-minute walk once a week, begin your program with very slow, easy, gentle walks until you reach these criteria.

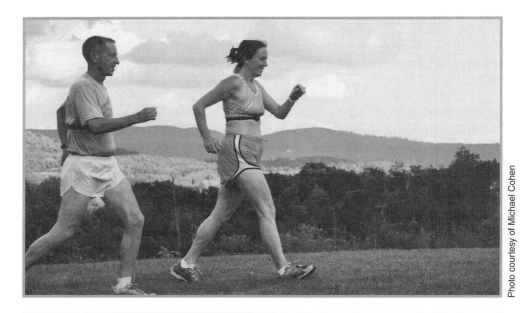

Photo courtesy of Michael Cohen

Using a heart rate monitor while you walk is a good way to measure your training level and optimize your intensity.

The following program is an individualized, structured plan that you can use to take your walking fitness to higher levels. Use your heart rate monitor to make sure your effort is hard enough to reach the quality needed to improve, but more important, to be sure that you do not try so hard that you overtrain and come down with a case of shin splints or worse.

Classifying Your Current Fitness Level

Before you can get a driver's license, you need to learn to make a car move where you want it to by practicing under proper supervision. Then you must take the exam to earn your license. At this point, you should have your learner's permit and have had plenty of practice. Now you need to take a test to determine your current state of fitness. This will help you pick the appropriate level of workout as your starting point.

Carefully look over the outline of the following test to make sure you understand all the instructions. Remember to wear a watch or take a stopwatch so you can time yourself. Also, wear your heart rate monitor to see how high your heart rate goes when you walk this time trial mile. Strap on your heart rate monitor, reset your stopwatch to zero, take a deep breath, and head for the track.

While doing the test, check your heart rate monitor every minute. Expect a fairly even, steady increase in the numbers, but be aware that the highest number may not be right at the finish of the test if you get tired and have to slow down before the end.

1-Mile Walking Test

1. Find a track or measure a flat trail with a smooth surface. On a standard track, one lap is 1/4 of a mile, so for 1 mile you will walk four laps. Use the inside lane. If you don't have access to a track, measure a route using your car's odometer. This method may not be quite as accurate but it will be close enough for this test.

2. Warm up with several minutes of easy walking and stretching.

3. Start the stopwatch and begin to walk 1 mile. Don't start too fast. Use a steady pace that makes you feel you are pushing hard. As you near the 1-mile mark, pick up the pace and finish strong. Stop the stopwatch. After the test, you should feel a little winded, but you shouldn't be exhausted.

4. Cool down with a few minutes of easy walking. Compare your time to table 9.1 to determine your walking classification.

If you met the prerequisites noted earlier, you likely are already in the health category. If you qualified in the fitness category, use the level 1 program to build a better base of endurance. If you reached the athletic category, start at level 2. Level 2 will be especially stimulating for your muscular and respiratory systems because it develops your stamina.

TABLE 9.1 Walking Classification Based on 1-Mile Walking Test Result

Men (in min)	Women (in min)	Walking classification
>16	>17	Health
13–16	14–17	Fitness
<13	<14	Athletic

Determining Your Walking Maximum Heart Rate

We have to admit that walkers present a bit of a conundrum when it comes to testing for MHR. Estimating MHR through the methods described in chapter 2, page 24, isn't very reliable. For other sports and exercise activities, it is standard practice to base target heart rates on percentages of MHR identified as the athlete runs up a steep incline on a treadmill at a high rate of speed. However, it is virtually impossible to walk to your MHR without the test constituting cruel and unusual punishment because low-intensity walking workouts inadequately challenge the muscular and respiratory systems

1-mile Walking Test adapted from *Fitness Walking*, 2nd edition, by Therese Iknoian, 2005, Human Kinetics, Inc., page 13.

for such a high-stress test. Even so, you need to test yourself somehow to calculate your target heart rates. The customized test described here is still intense and should be attempted only with permission from your doctor.

The Connolly-Benson stress test for walkers requires a treadmill. Before starting the test, check your heart rate monitor for possible interference from the electrical console of the treadmill. If your numbers are erratic and make no sense, you may have to ask a friend to hold your receiver off to the side out of the range of the treadmill's control board.

Start by walking for 3 minutes at 3 miles per hour (4.8 km/h) to warm up. Raise the elevation 1 percent and walk for 1 minute. Raise the elevation another 1 percent and walk another minute. Continue raising the elevation 1 percent every minute. Do not hold on to the guardrails or hand bar. Carefully monitor your heart rate a couple of times per minute. When the combination of the speed and the incline make it impossible for you to keep up, double-check your heart rate, note this number, and then slow down the belt speed and decrease the elevation. Walk for several minutes to cool down. For walking purposes, you have established a maximum heart rate.

Your walking MHR is an important given that will allow us to use the classic design of a scientific experiment for your progression in this program. Your goal will be to get in better shape by walking farther without exceeding your upper heart rate limit. The long-term variable of the experiment is the period of time it takes you to cover the given distance without exceeding your upper heart rate limit. As your endurance improves, the walks will become easier and your heart will not have to work as hard, thus allowing you to walk faster. Your current fitness level is the short-term variable to measure if you can keep the other workout elements, such as pace and terrain, constant as givens. Admittedly, the elements that influence your heart rate on workout days, such as the temperature, the wind, surface flatness, your degree of recovery from previous workouts, and your stress level, can vary from day to day. By not exceeding your upper heart rate target, you will ensure that you stay in the endurance- and stamina-development zones.

Practical scientists deal with these varying conditions by using finagled factors. You, too, may have to be a bit broad-minded and play with your walking speed to adjust for conditions when you work out. To keep within your target zone, you may have to slow down on bad days or speed up on good days. Look at the big picture to make sure that your workout heart rates, not your speed, are constant over a week or two.

In two to three weeks, you'll notice that your heart rate response at the same walking speed decreases. The goal is to track that slowly decreasing number of beats per minute as you get in better shape. You will do that by using the goal time of your workouts as another given. During each progression, you will repeat the same workouts until you can cover the time of each progression without exceeding your upper target heart rate.

In level 1, you'll improve your endurance by doing more reps with your light body weight as you walk longer.

Determining Your Walking Training Zones

Your lower target heart rate is 50 percent of your walking MHR, and your upper target heart rate is 75 percent of your walking MHR. As long as you are within that range, but definitely not exceeding the upper limit, you will be safe from the pace police. Your challenge is to walk fast enough to at least reach your lower target heart rate and then fast and far enough without exceeding your upper target heart rate. These target heart rates will be givens in your fitness measurement.

Another given will be to go for the prescribed longer time than you did on the test. Your primary variable will be your pace per mile. Following our heart rate fartlek protocol, you will change your pace as needed to stay within your target zones.

You will do each workout within three heart rate zones: a lower zone, a recovery zone, and an upper zone.

1. Your lower target heart rate is 50 percent of your MHR from the tread-mill test (page 117). This is the beats per minute you should reach when you start timing your workouts. By the end of a 5-minute warm-up walk, you must be going fast enough to approach this number. Keep in mind that we're looking for a realistic number that you'd see at a casual stroll effort.

2. Your recovery heart rate is 65 to 70 percent of your walking MHR. Use this target if you start to exceed your upper target. Just slow down until your heart rate drops into this zone. Then, pick up the pace again and go farther until you again start to exceed your upper limit.

3. Your upper target heart rate is always 75 percent of the walking MHR identified during the treadmill stress test (page 117). If you doubt that number, perform the test again and recalculate your target heart rates.

The progressions with each program level are designed to challenge you by making you walk for more minutes. When you reach your upper target heart rate, slow down and let your heart rate drop until it hits the recovery rate; then pick it up again. Eventually, you will cover the entire workout without reaching your upper target. When you achieve that, you're ready to graduate to the next progression.

Choosing a Training Program

Deciding where to begin depends on how you scored on the 1-mile walking test. Level 1 workouts will expand your base of aerobic endurance. Level 2 workouts will improve your stamina. Those are the first two phases of conditioning for every endurance-based sport. The fitness developed here may bring you to a point at which you decide to try something more challenging. If so, you'll be able to springboard off a fairly good base of overall fitness.

Progressions are labeled alphabetically by level of difficulty. As you move from one progression to the next, the conditioning responses you're seeking will require longer and longer efforts.

The programs that follow are based on the experimental model discussed earlier, with upper target heart rate zone always being the primary given that you should not exceed during the workout. Variables are time, distance, and pace. For example, at level 1 you are given a period of time to walk at whatever pace feels biomechanically optimal. That pace should be close to what you maintained during the 1-mile test if you did not need a week off, massage therapy, or medical treatment to recover from the strains to your musculoskeletal system.

During a workout, if the additional distance causes your heart rate to exceed your upper limit, you will need an interval of slower pace and easier effort to drop to your target recovery number of 70 percent MHR. Obviously, the more time you spend going slowly during recovery, the shorter the total distance will be that you'll cover during the prescribed time. As your fitness improves, you will need less time for recovery, and you'll go farther in the same amount of time for each progression. Eventually, your endurance will reach an optimal stage at which point you will be enjoying a healthy level of cardiovascular fitness. Once you are able to walk the programmed number of minutes at the top speed at which you are biomechanically comfortable, your reward will be to see how much easier walking becomes by tracking both your morning resting heart rate and your heart rate at the end of the workout. You'll be able to walk at the same speed at a lower heart rate, indicating improved fitness. When time is the experimental given, then your improved fitness is the variable to measure.

The walking program levels are based on your tested degree of fitness. The progressive workouts in each level will incrementally take your physical fitness to higher levels. The progressions are based on more minutes of exercise. Use your recent history as well as your score from the 1-mile walking test to find a reasonable starting point. You will notice as you review the progressions that they do not require you to follow them for a certain number of weeks. How long you stay with a particular progression will depend on your heart rate response. When you can complete the entire workout without exceeding your upper target heart rate, it is time to go to the next progression. That's the beauty of this protocol: it offers a totally individualized program. This means that you have the most customized possible answer to the "What about me?" question.

Level 1

The level 1 workouts feature a range of minutes based on your time from the 1-mile walking test. Because the fastest time for a male in the fitness category is 13 minutes and the fastest time for a female is 16 minutes, we've used a target time of 30 minutes to start our progressions. The weekly long walk is 10 minutes longer. However, to customize the time ranges based on your current fitness level, you can simply double your test time. This will help you reach the goal of improving your endurance as soon as possible.

Start each workout with an easy 5-minute stroll that slowly increases your heart rate to your lower target (50 percent of your walking MHR). When you can do these workouts without exceeding your upper target, go to the next progression.

Progression A

Monday through Friday

Walk 30 minutes on three or four of these days.

Saturday or Sunday

Walk 40 minutes on one of these days.

Progression B

Monday through Friday

Walk 35 minutes on four of these days.

Saturday or Sunday

Walk 45 minutes on one of these days.

Progression C

Monday through Friday

Walk 40 minutes on four or five of these days.

Saturday or Sunday

Walk 50 minutes on one of these days.

After completing progression C, you may choose to continue this level 1 routine to enjoy a healthy level of cardiovascular health and long-term weight control. Simply stay at progression C in level 1. However, if you are interested in a higher level of physical fitness, repeat the 1-mile walking test to see if you can reach the athletic category. If so, and you wish to work harder and get healthier, proceed to level 2.

Level 2

In the level 2 program, you will face hard days of higher intensity that will improve your cardiorespiratory fitness. There is only one practical way to elevate your breathing and heart rate to stamina levels while walking: going vertical. Yes, that means going uphill. This increases your resistance to gravity and enables you to achieve a major increase in your working heart rate. Choose stairs, stadium steps, hills, or incline settings on a treadmill.

The goal of the level 2 program is to develop stamina by increasing the intensity of exercise. To reduce the risk of injury and overtraining, you will need to follow the classic hard/easy workout pattern that allows recovery from higher-intensity workouts by separating them with off or easy days. You also may have to warm up an extra 5 minutes before your workout on hard days. On recovery days, the closer you keep your effort to the lower target, the more effective your recovery will be.

On the easy recovery days, walk for at least 20 minutes but not longer than 30 minutes, keeping your heart rate between 50 and 60 percent of your walking MHR.

Before you start the progressions, choose one of the patterns of hard/easy workouts shown in table 9.2. Choose your pattern based on which weekend day you prefer for your longer walk.

Both patterns require flexibility. Feel free to switch the off and easy days as needed. However, if you have to miss a hard day, do not make it up the next day and wind up doing two hard days back to back. Either skip the missed workout and stick with the pattern, or move everything back a day. In the long term, there are no penalties for doing back-to-back easy days. However, the injury fairy may get after you for trying to do two hard days in a row.

Level 2 workouts also use our experimental format. Each progression has a given number of uphill trips to your upper target heart rate in whatever time it takes to hit the target interspersed with intervals of downhill or flat recovery times to drop to your lower target heart rate. The time it takes you to hit the upper target depends on the steepness of the surface. This provides a great deal of flexibility: less incline means a longer time to reach the target heart rate; more incline means a shorter time to reach the target heart rate. But please stick with the same incline during the three progressions because you must measure how long it takes initially to reach your upper target. Proof of your improved fitness will be the increasingly longer time it takes to reach that target.

Your recovery interval times between repeated uphill trips will vary as you become more fatigued with each uphill trip.

This program assumes that you will have improved your stamina to an adequate degree by the end of the third progression. To prove it to yourself, see how much farther you walk during the 1-mile walking test.

TABLE 9.2 Level 2 Hard/Easy Patterns

Weekly pattern 1						
Sun.	**Mon.**	**Tues.**	**Wed.**	**Thurs.**	**Fri.**	**Sat.**
Long walk	Easy	Hard	Off or easy	Hard	Easy	Off
Weekly pattern 2						
Sun.	**Mon.**	**Tues.**	**Wed.**	**Thurs.**	**Fri.**	**Sat.**
Off	Hard	Easy	Hard	Easy	Off	Long walk

Calculate your new upper target heart rate by using 85 percent of your walking MHR as discovered during the treadmill test (page 117). Your new target heart rate is appropriate if you start to fail the talk test just as you reach the target number. You should be huffing and puffing enough to kill your enthusiasm for saying even a quick yes or no.

Time is a variable and depends on the steepness of the incline. Once you reach your upper target (85 percent of your walking MHR), walk back down the incline or lower the treadmill incline setting until your heart rate drops to 70 percent MHR. Before and after each workout, walk easily for 10 minutes to warm up and cool down.

Progression A

Hard Days

Walk up the incline of your choice until you reach your upper target heart rate. Time is a variable and depends on the steepness of the incline. Once you reach your upper target (85 percent of your walking MHR), walk back down the incline or lower the treadmill incline setting until your heart rate drops to 70 percent MHR. Do this twice. Before and after each workout, walk easily for 10 minutes to warm up and cool down.

Easy Days

On recovery days, walk for at least 20 minutes but not longer than 30 minutes, keeping your heart rate between 50 and 60 percent of your walking MHR.

Long Day

Once a week, walk for 50 minutes without exceeding 75 percent of your walking MHR. Your time goal does not include whatever easier, slower pace you need to warm up and cool down.

Follow progression A for two weeks. After the two weeks, take a recovery week without any hills. During the recovery week, walk 40 minutes four or five times Monday through Friday and 50 minutes once on the weekend.

Progression B

Hard Days

Walk up the incline of your choice until you reach your upper target heart rate. Time is a variable and depends on the steepness of the incline. Once you reach your upper target (85 percent of your walking MHR), walk back down the incline or lower the treadmill incline setting until your heart rate drops to 70 percent MHR. Do this four times. Before and after each workout, walk easily for 10 minutes to warm up and cool down.

Easy Days

On recovery days, walk for 30 minutes, keeping your heart rate between 50 and 60 percent of your walking MHR.

Long Day

Once a week, walk for 55 minutes without exceeding 75 percent of your walking MHR. Your time goal does not include whatever easier, slower pace you need to warm up and cool down.

Follow progression B for two weeks. After the two weeks, take a recovery week without any hills. During the recovery week, walk 40 minutes four or five times Monday through Friday and 50 minutes once on the weekend.

Progression C

Hard Days

Walk up the incline of your choice until you reach your upper target heart rate. Time is a variable and depends on the steepness of the incline. Once you reach your upper target (85 percent of your walking MHR), walk back down the incline or lower the treadmill incline setting until your heart rate drops to 70 percent MHR. Do this six times. Before and after each workout, walk easily for 10 minutes to warm up and cool down.

Easy Days

On recovery days, walk for 30 minutes, keeping your heart rate between 50 and 60 percent of your walking MHR.

Long Day

Once a week, walk for 60 minutes without exceeding 75 percent of your walking MHR. Your time goal does not include whatever easier, slower pace you need to warm up and cool down.

Follow progression C for two weeks. After the two weeks, take a recovery week without any hills. During the recovery week, walk 40 minutes four or five times Monday through Friday and 50 minutes once on the weekend.

Repeat progression C as long as you wish, but be sure to take a recovery week after each two-week period of hill work. If your pattern is interrupted for any reason and you miss two weeks or more, do at least one week of level 1 training before resuming the level 2 workouts at a lower progression.

Continuing Your Training

After completing level 2, you will be a very fit walker with a strong cardio-respiratory system. Enjoy your higher level of physical fitness as you decide whether you want to try the challenge of jogging and running. If so, read on.

CHAPTER 10

Jogging and Running

Nothing enhances compliance with an exercise program more than convenience, and few activities are more convenient than jogging or running. Just slip on your sneakers and jump on the treadmill or head out the door. Compliance also is enhanced when you have a successful, systematic approach to training and a structured program to follow.

The jogging and running programs in this chapter take into account the health improvements from exercise that stimulates the cardiovascular, cardiorespiratory, and musculoskeletal systems. Unfortunately, as you seek to improve health and fitness, the risk of injury or illness also gradually increases.

Therefore, for your body's sake, you need to understand the effects your workouts might have on your health as well as your ability to compete in races. The American College of Sports Medicine, not surprisingly, believes that exercise is good medicine. However, those docs also know that although jacking up the intensity and volume of workouts can be very beneficial, those harder workouts also have health risks. The good news is that you can minimize those risks with the individualization that our monitored and well-planned training offers.

Developing either recreational or competitive levels of fitness takes time. Getting in better shape may take weeks or months as gravity's resistance to movement when you exercise stimulates your body to make the desired improvements in your fitness. In previous chapters, we discussed the physiological, biochemical, and biomechanical changes associated with this process for all types of exercise and activities. This chapter focuses on making those changes happen by jogging and running.

The programs outlined here are designed for people who already have a base level of fitness and want to use their time and energy effectively. If your most recent medical exam confirms that your risk factors are low, if you have been jogging for 20 minutes three or four times week, and if you can jog at least 30 minutes in one workout, you qualify to use the level 1 jogging program. If this does not describe you, get approval from your doctor. Then take several months of very easy, slow jogging and walking to reach these entry qualifications. If you already run more frequently or longer, be sure to take the $\dot{V}O_2$max test on the next page to classify your current level of fitness and choose a running program from levels 2 or 3 based on your current fitness level and your running goals.

Jogging is an effective exercise for weight control, but it carries a slightly higher risk of overuse injuries because of the distances required to really burn off fat. Be especially sensitive to aches and pains from sore, stiff muscles and joints. Do not try to push through the pain. What athletes refer to as the pain barrier is the total body fatigue and exhaustion that comes from going for peak performances at 100 percent effort. Pains in your muscles, ligaments, tendons, and bones, however, are symptoms of injuries and are not to be ignored. Don't just mask them with over-the-counter painkillers such as aspirin and NSAIDS. Back off, rest up, and then resume when the symptoms have gone away. Remember that 60 percent of your maximum heart rate (MHR) is your lower target, and 75 percent MHR is your upper limit. Everything in between is productive, although with slightly different benefits at either end.

Joggers and runners have one very important training objective in common: to improve endurance by training in the zone of 60 to 75 percent MHR. For many joggers, good cardiovascular health, weight management, and that intangible feeling of well-being are the major goals. For competitive runners, endurance training is simply to build the foundation of aerobic fitness to support the next stages of conditioning. A runner's training pattern needs to be more comprehensive and include some workouts that are unnecessary for joggers.

The level 1 program for joggers features a series of progressions based solely on heart rate targets to improve endurance. You need not overdo it by working harder than necessary to enjoy a good level of endurance. (That may be good news if you

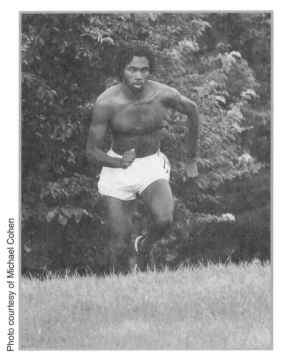

Photo courtesy of Michael Cohen

Joggers and runners both seek to build a good base of endurance. Runners then build on this base to reach higher levels of conditioning.

have been working harder than necessary.) If you only want to jog enough to build fitness and manage weight, you will need to take the MHR test on page 129, but you do not need to determine your $\dot{V}O_2$max or anaerobic threshold because the level 1 program does not involve efforts at those levels. After determining your MHR, you can move on to the programs that begin on page 131.

The level 2 program is for you if you are a recreational runner who wants to participate in 5Ks, 10Ks, half marathons, and full marathons and finish smiling but are not looking to be competitive. If you want to be competitive in 5Ks, 10Ks, half marathons, or full marathons, or are seeking peak personal record performances, the level 3 programs are for you.

To answer the "What about me?" question, you need to do a little self-evaluating and calculating. First, you need to classify your current level of fitness. Second, you need to find your jogging or running MHR. Third, you need to calculate your current anaerobic threshold. (If you are interested in the level 1 jogging program only and meet the criteria described earlier, you don't need to classify your current level of fitness or determine your anaerobic threshold.) This information will help you calculate your target heart rate zones and build the best training program for you.

Classifying Your Current Fitness Level

If you are a recreational or competitive runner, use this simple, modified treadmill test to predict your oxygen uptake capacity, or $\dot{V}O_2$max. Use tables 10.1, 10.2, and 10.3 to interpret the results and determine your level of training. To get the most reliable and valid results, taper your training for a few days before taking the test.

Start the test at a very slow speed to warm up. If you find the starting speed of the test—6 miles per hour (9.6 km/h) at a 2 percent grade—fairly easy, start with that speed and build the warm-up into the test protocol.

Run on the treadmill at the identified speed for each stage (see table 10.1). Adjust the speed every 2 minutes until you can no longer complete a stage. The last stage you complete is your ending stage, or workload. Use this stage to classify your fitness level and calculate your $\dot{V}O_2$max. If you want to collect MHR data simultaneously, wear your heart rate monitor and record your heart rate at the end of the test.

This prediction of your maximum oxygen consumption is based on a formula developed by the American College of Sports Medicine (*ACSM's Guidelines for Testing and Prescription, fifth edition.* Baltimore: Williams & Wilkins, 1995, pp. 278-283). Table 10.1 lists the approximate $\dot{V}O_2$ needed to run at this speed and grade over this time period. Once you have your ending $\dot{V}O_2$max, look for your fitness classification in table 10.2 (if you are male) or table 10.3 (if you are female), using the maximum oxygen consumption value you achieved. Your program level is determined by matching your $\dot{V}O_2$max score from table 10.1 with the data in either table 10.2 or table 10.3. Find the line on the table that corresponds to your age.

TABLE 10.1 Prediction of $\dot{V}O_2$max Based on Treadmill Running Times

Stage	Duration (min)	Speed (mph)	Grade (%)	$\dot{V}O_2$max (ml/kg/min)
0	2:00	6.0	2	38.54
1	2:00	6.5	2	41.46
2	2:00	7.0	2	44.38
3	2:00	7.5	2	47.30
4	2:00	8.0	2	50.22
5	2:00	8.5	2	53.14
6	2:00	9.0	2	56.06
7	2:00	9.5	2	58.98
8	2:00	10.0	2	61.90
9	2:00	10.5	2	64.82
10	2:00	11.0	2	67.70
11	2:00	11.5	2	70.60

TABLE 10.2 Fitness Classifications Based on $\dot{V}O_2$max Results: Male Athletes

Age	Poor	Fair	Average	Good	Excellent
15–19	≤52	53–57	58–65	66–69	≥70
20–29	≤52	53–59	60–69	70–77	≥78
30–39	≤47	48–53	54–62	63–71	≥72
40–49	≤39	40–43	44–55	56–63	≥64
50–59	≤31	32–37	38–51	52–57	≥58
60–69	≤22	23–30	31–42	43–54	≥55
	Level 1		Level 2		Level 3

Note: Classifications reflect conditioning status for endurance athletes. Data for nonathletes would be much lower.

TABLE 10.3 Fitness Classifications Based on $\dot{V}O_2$max Results: Female Athletes

Age	Poor	Fair	Average	Good	Excellent
15–19	≤48	49–54	55–61	62–67	≥68
20–29	≤49	50–54	55–62	63–71	≥72
30–39	≤39	40–49	50–55	56–64	≥65
40–49	≤28	29–40	41–48	49–59	≥60
50–59	≤19	20–28	29–40	41–50	≥51
60–69	≤7	8–14	15–25	26–41	≥42
	Level 1		Level 2		Level 3

Note: Classifications reflect conditioning status for endurance athletes. Data for nonathletes would be much lower.

For example, let's say you are a 30-year-old female and you complete stage 4. Your predicted $\dot{V}O_2$max is 50.22 ml/kg/min. This would give you a rating of average. We suggest you start with a level 2 training program.

If you score at level 3, you may immediately start your heart rate–monitored workouts at the advanced stage of conditioning, beginning on page 136. However, we strongly urge you to review the level 1 and level 2 programs to ensure that your endurance, stamina, and economy are sufficiently developed to allow you to sustain a serious season of competition and to peak at the right time.

Determining Your Running Maximum Heart Rate

Both maximum and target heart rates are sport specific. Because your workouts will be based on target heart rate zones, we provide two runner-specific tests for determining your running MHR. A formal treadmill stress test in a cardiologist's office or physiology lab is the best way to determine your true MHR, but most of us don't have access to such tests. The tests outlined in this book provide good estimates and so are good alternatives.

The first test, described in chapter 2 (page 24), is best for those with more speed than endurance. Surviving the three efforts of very high intensity and high speed without significant muscle stiffness and soreness requires a very good level of fitness.

The second test is better suited for those with more endurance and patience, and a lower level of fitness. The protocol for this second test is based on the design for a graded treadmill maximum stress test. The difference is that it doesn't require a treadmill. It has the same graded increments of increasing speed and intensity, but without the steep incline at the end. Here is how you do it:

Find a 400-meter running track. Dress to run, and put on your heart rate monitor. Begin at the end of a straightaway at the start of a curve. Cover eight laps as described. Check your working heart rate every 200 meters.

Lap 1: Walk an easy lap at your normal walking pace.

Lap 2: Walk faster for another lap at close to a marching pace.

Lap 3: Jog one lap at the slowest jogging pace you can manage.

Lap 4: Break into an easy, slow run at a conversational pace for one lap.

Lap 5: Run hard enough to lightly huff and puff at a short-sentences pace.

Lap 6: Run hard enough to huff and puff hard and fast enough to lose your desire to answer even a yes or no question.

Laps 7 and 8: Run faster on each of the last two laps, increasing the pace and effort at the start of each curve so the last half lap is an all-out, maximum effort.

Remember to check your heart rate every 200 meters. Expect a steady, incremental increase at the end of each of the first six laps. Carefully read your heart rate at least four times during the last two laps.

When you are running hard and wearing the monitor on your wrist like a watch, seeing the numbers can be difficult. Try holding the monitor in your hand and lifting it in front of your face as you run. To do so, buckle the wrist strap and make a loop. Slip your middle two fingers through the loop. Cradle the top and bottom of the face between your thumb and first finger so it is in position for you to read when you swing your arm forward in its natural motion.

Do not stop dead in your tracks when you are finished. After the final lap, walk around while double-checking your heart rate. The highest number you see during or right after the test is probably within several beats per minute of your true maximum. For our purposes, that is close enough.

Before trying either of these tests, be sure your doctor has cleared you for exercise. If you have any doubts about the validity of the test, repeat it every week until you are satisfied with the results. Just remember that your own MHR may be way over or under your predicted MHR from the age-adjusted formula.

Determining Your Running Anaerobic Threshold

A runner in good competitive shape will have an anaerobic threshold (AT) between 85 and 90 percent MHR, according to most experts. Anaerobic threshold reflects your body's ability to take in, distribute, and use oxygen and depends on the capacities and the fitness of your respiratory, circulatory, and muscular systems. These three systems, although interrelated, enjoy different levels of capacity for work at the same time. This means that AT is a rather fluid component of fitness and that there is a direct correlation between your AT and your heart rate. If your AT is below lousy, your heart rate will be lower than the 85 percent that you would expect. Equally surprising can be how heavy and hard your breathing will be at such low heart rates.

This can explained by using an example of a runner whose training has been strictly focused on endurance. Because almost all of the work is done at highly aerobic effort in the 60 to 75 percent target heart rate zone, the cardiovascular system gets lots of work, but the easy effort hardly challenges the respiratory or muscular systems. As a result, when the workouts get more difficult, those latter two systems are not in very good shape, although the heart has gotten much stronger as revealed in the significant drop in resting heart rate.

After a long layoff or lots of easy distance work, you may find yourself breathing really hard at an apparently easy and low heart rate such as, say, 73 percent MHR. You probably are now training at your current AT. Not to worry. Lots of stamina training will raise your AT to 80 to 85 percent, and economy workouts will take it up to as high as 90 percent.

Another useful, but not as accurate, way to determine your current AT is to run until the effort feels difficult and you are huffing and puffing too fast to talk in anything but one-word sentences. Although this pace is uncomfortable, you can sustain it for 2 to 3 miles (3.2 to 4.8 km). This is a rough estimate of your pace and heart rate at your current AT.

With that description and the previous discussion in mind, take your heart rate monitor out for a workout. Jog slowly for several minutes and then pick up the pace while frequently monitoring your heart rate. Note your heart rate when your perceived effort reaches the one-word-sentence stage. For all practical purposes, this is your current AT. Rest assured that your AT is a fluid point along a continuum of beats per minute over a wide range and that it basically reveals the shape you're in. Your perception of the effort will stay the same, but as you get in better shape, your heart rate will go higher while the pace gets faster.

Determining Your Running Training Zones

Once you have a reliable estimate of your MHR, you can determine your training zones. Remember that training zones are sport specific; they may vary for other activities. Use your estimated MHR and the target heart-rate calculator on pages 25 and 27 to determine the beats per minute for each zone:

Long, endurance-building runs: 60–75% MHR

Easy, recovery jogs: 65–70% MHR

Maximal recovery and taper jogs: 60–65% MHR

Stamina runs: 75–85% MHR

Economy runs: 85–95% MHR

Speed and power runs: 95–100% MHR

Record your training zones based on these percentages, and use them to plan and monitor your training.

Choosing a Training Program

This section presents a set of idealized training programs that feature workouts to develop all four components of fitness—endurance, stamina, economy, and speed—through each of the four training phases that progressively develop those components. Level 1 is for joggers who wish to build endurance and enjoy better health and weight control. Level 2 workouts develop endurance and stamina for recreational runners who wish to finish 5Ks, 10Ks, half marathons, and full marathons but not compete at an elite level. Level 3 builds economy, speed, and power where appropriate for racing runners who aspire to compete against the clock to set personal records and beat other competitors in 5Ks, 10Ks, half marathons, and full marathons. Level 3 features workouts to take racing runners down the home stretch as fast as hungry cheetahs, helping them peak at the right time of the season.

Level 1: Jogging to Build Endurance

It might appear a bit exaggerated, but the range of 60 percent MHR as your lower target heart rate and 75 percent MHR as your upper limit is valid. It's true that the lower end is best for maintaining endurance and the upper end is best for developing endurance. Slightly different benefits occur at either end, but everything in between is productive.

This program uses the scientific format of givens, or controls, and a variable. In each progression, the stated duration of the workout and the frequency of workouts in a week are givens. The most important given is the set of target heart rates. That allows you to track your improving fitness as a variable by measuring how much distance you cover each day. For example, if you use a running track, you might cover only three or four laps during your first 30-minute workout. Three or four weeks later, you might be able to complete five or six laps in 30 minutes because you can go longer before reaching your upper limit. You'll spend less time walking because your heart rate will drop faster into your recovery zone.

If you prefer to run on the street instead of a track, use a landmark, such as a neighbor's mailbox, to note where you finish the first time. Soon you'll be going past that mailbox to the gas station on the corner. You could also break the duration of the workout into half periods and then note how much farther past the starting line you go as you return from the turnaround point day after day, week after week.

The number of weeks it takes you to accomplish each progression is the ending variable. In short, you are measuring both short- and long-term improvements in your fitness.

Your jogging pace and how much walking you have to do to recover once (and if) you exceed your upper heart rate limit will determine how much distance you cover during the specified time. The beauty of using our heart rate fartlek protocol is that you will answer the "What about me?" question because the variable reflects your current level of fitness.

Even if you are already doing what seems to be more mileage than is covered in progression A, follow it as an introduction to using target heart rate zones. If you are in better shape, you'll simply graduate to progression B sooner.

Progression A

Use the first 5 minutes of your workout to warm up by gently getting to and then not exceeding 65 percent MHR. Plan to use the last 5 minutes to jog or walk your heart rate down to well below 60 percent as a cool-down These 10 minutes count as part of the total time of the workout.

Monday Through Friday

Jog 30 minutes of heart rate fartlek on three weekdays. Jog until your heart rate reaches 75 percent MHR; then walk it down to 60 percent. Repeat as needed for the 30 minutes.

Saturday or Sunday

Jog 40 minutes of heart rate fartlek on one weekend day. Jog until your heart rate reaches 75 percent MHR; then walk it down to 60 percent.

Repeat this pattern for as many weeks as necessary until you are able to cover the entire period without exceeding 75 percent MHR and without walking. Feel free to cut back the number of minutes by 10 to 20 percent for the week if you start noticing that you are not going as far during your workouts. You may be overtraining. Your legs will tell you. Listen to them and don't bravely try to follow the plan to the minute.

Progression B

Use the first 5 minutes of your workout to warm up by gently getting to and then not exceeding 65 percent MHR. Plan to use the last 5 minutes to jog or walk your heart rate down to well below 60 percent as a cool-down. These 10 minutes count as part of the total time of the workout.

Monday Through Friday

Jog 30 minutes of heart rate fartlek on four weekdays. Jog until your heart rate reaches 75 percent MHR; then walk it down to 60 percent.

Saturday or Sunday

Jog 50 minutes of heart rate fartlek on one weekend day. Jog until your heart rate reaches 75 percent MHR; then walk it down to 60 percent.

Repeat this pattern for as many weeks as necessary until you are able to cover the entire period without exceeding 75 percent MHR and without walking. Carefully monitor your legs for any signs of chronic fatigue such as dead or heavy legs. Cut back the number of minutes if you need to.

Progression C

Use the first 10 minutes of your workout to warm up by gently getting to and then not exceeding 65 percent MHR. Plan to use the last 5 minutes to jog or walk your heart rate down to well below 60 percent as a cool-down. These 15 minutes count as part of the total time of the workout.

Monday Through Friday

Take a day off on Monday, Wednesday, or Friday. On the other two days (Monday, Wednesday, or Friday), jog for 30 minutes without exceeding 75 percent MHR. On Tuesday and Thursday, jog for 45 minutes, staying in the 70 to 75 percent MHR zone.

Saturday and Sunday

On Saturday, rest up for a long jog on Sunday by jogging for 20 minutes at 60 to 65 percent MHR. On Sunday, increase the length of the weekend workout to 60 minutes without exceeding 75 percent MHR and without walking.

If your legs get heavy and your pace slows down as a result of overtraining, go back to progression B for a week. To lower the risk of overtraining, make every fourth week a recovery week and follow the progression A pattern.

At this point, your endurance should be adequate for all practical purposes, your weight well controlled, and your good looks at an all-time best. Feel free to mix and match your workouts into different patterns to add some variety. Consider increasing your fitness and advancing to a recreational running level. If you would like to become a recreational runner, go back and take the $\dot{V}O_2$max and anaerobic threshold tests, and then read on.

Level 2: Running for Recreation

For these programs, heart rate zones are used as givens. This allows you to track a response that is completely individualized to your level of fitness and ability. Each workout level switches around the variables as required to achieve each level of conditioning.

Even if you are sure of your current fitness level and qualify to start with a level 2 or level 3 program, please remember not to go too fast too soon. You have to crawl before you can walk and walk before you can run.

Use your current fitness level and the result from your $\dot{V}O_2$max test to pick a category and starting level. Don't be afraid to start low to build a new base of aerobic endurance. This might be the ideal time to do so.

The program in table 10.4 will help you develop your fitness so you can finish a 5K, 10K, half marathon, or marathon with a smile but no concern with place or time. You may think the program seems short on the total weekly volume. However, it does not include any extra minutes you add warming up or cooling down before and after your harder workouts. Your warm-ups and cool-downs might add as much as 30 to 45 more minutes per week. Do at least a 10-minute warm-up jog and then jog for 5 minutes to cool down after the workout.

If you find the total minutes per week a bit daunting, rest assured that the minutes on your easy days include whatever time you spend warming up and cooling down. However, the harder days require a 10-minute jog to warm up and a 5-minute jog to cool down. If that pushes your weekly running total too high for comfort, adjust the minutes downward by 15 to 20 percent or more, especially if you see signs of overtraining.

The program also features some stamina training, so it does not strictly follow the principle of the four phases of training. If your endurance capacity is inadequate to attempt this mixed pattern, go back and work through the level 1 jogging program. When you can complete it, move up to level 2.

This progression demonstrates how to get in shape to be ready to get in better shape. This endurance training model works well for all four distances, but runners who wish to get in competitive shape need to follow separate programs with their distinctive mix of higher-intensity workouts. Ironically, those who choose the shorter-distance races will have to work harder at higher percentages of MHR, whereas half marathoners and marathoners will have to work harder by running more but at lower intensities.

TABLE 10.4 Level 2: 24-Week Program for Recreational Runners (5K, 10K, Half Marathon, and Full Marathon)

Week	Phase	Minutes per week*	Mon.	Tues.	Wed.	Thurs.	Fri.	Sat.	Sun.
1	I	150:00	Off	25:00 A	30:00 A	25:00 A	Off	20:00 A	50:00 B
2	I	165:00	Off	35:00 A	25:00 A	35:00 A	Off	28:00 A	57:00 B
3	I	180:00	Off	30:00 A	25:00 A	25:00 C	Off	35:00 A	65:00 B
4	I and II	195:00	Off	30:00 A	25:00 C	35:00 C	Off	35:00 A	70:00 B
5	I and II	215:00	Off	35:00 C	30:00 A	4 × D	Off	45:00 A	75:00 B
6	I and II	> 155:00	45:00 A	3 × D	60:00 A	Off	25:00 A	Off	5K
7	I and II	200:00	Off	30:00 C	30:00 A	3 × D	Off	45:00 A	70:00 B
8	I and II	225:00	Off	4 × D	45:00 A	25:00 E	Off	50:00 A	80:00 B
9	I and II	250:00	Off	5 × D	50:00 A	25:00 E	Off	50:00 A	90:00 B
10	I and II	> 155:00	Off	45:00 A	3 × D	50:00 A	35:00 A	Off	10K
11	I	225:00	Off	30:00 A	45:00 A	30:00 A	Off	45:00 A	75:00 B
12	I and II	255:00	Off	40:00 A	6 × D	35:00 A	Off	45:00 A	90:00 B
13	I	290:00	Off	35:00 C	35:00 A	35:00 C	30:00 A	50:00 F	105:00 B
14	I and II	330:00	25:00 A	30:00 A	7 × D	30:00 A	40:00 A	30:00 F	120:00 B
15	I	250:00	Off	40:00 C	35:00 A	30:00 A	35:00 C	35:00 A	75:00 B
16	I and II	> 155:00	35:00 A	3 × D	50:00 A	25:00 A	Off	20:00 F	Half marathon
17	I	250:00	40:00 A	Off	50:00 A	40:00 A	Off	45:00 A	75:00 B
18	I	290:00	30:00 A	45:00 C	25:00 A	Off	40:00 C	50:00 A	100:00 B
19	I	340:00	35:00 A	55:00 C	30:00 A	20:00 A	45:00 C	40:00 A	125:00 B
20	I	390:00	30:00 A	65:00 C	30:00 A	30:00 A	50:00 C	35:00 F	150:00 B
21	I	440:00	45:00 A	75:00 C	40:00 A	Off	55:00 C	45:00 F	180:00 B
22	II	260:00	Off	60:00 C	45:00 A	Off	4 × D	30:00 F	90:00 B
23	II	> 170:00	Off	35:00 A	45:00 A	40:00 A	30:00 A	20:00 F	Full marathon
24	I	130:00	25:00 A	Off	30:00 A	Off	30:00 A	Off	45:00 A

*Minutes per week does not include time for races.

KEY

A: Easy effort at 65–70% MHR
B: Endurance-building long run at 60–75% MHR
C: Moderate effort, steady pace at 75–80% MHR
D: Number of 7:00 repeats at 80–85% MHR with 2:00 jog interval to less than 70% MHR
E: Tempo (nonstop running) at anaerobic threshold, 80–85% MHR
F: Very easy effort at 60–65% MHR

Level 3: Running to Compete

Level 3 training programs are not appropriate for beginners. These programs add training at intensities to improve economy so you'll be more competitive, and speed and power to prepare you for peak racing performances that set personal records. You need to have at least one full year of running experience and currently run at least 215 minutes per week at level 2. We'll use the same experimental model that prepared walkers in chapter 9 and joggers in level 1 of this chapter. Your exercising target heart rates and recovery target heart rates, as well as the length of the runs in minutes, will be the givens. The variable will be your pace.

In the true spirit of this book, every workout uses heart rate as the exclusive guide for determining paces. The beauty of this system is that your particular current fitness level, general ability, and goals won't matter. You will be doing the same workout as every other reader based on the universal principles of exercise science known to prepare athletes to perform successfully at their chosen events. The only difference is that some of the luckier ones will finish the workouts sooner, but everyone benefits equally with the same adaptations.

Before you peek ahead at the training programs, please read this section explaining their rationales. The programs give a week-by-week schedule of the big picture for the entire training period. The patterns give a micropicture of each daily workout. The programs progress by starting with higher volume and lower intensity and then gradually raise intensity while decreasing volume. We hope this approach will help you avoid all the dreaded overuse injuries and the common mistake of overtraining, which commonly results from going too fast or too far too soon.

Each week has a goal of running X number of minutes, which you can translate into miles or kilometers, in Y number of days. We suggest that you run five or six days per week maximum. Please note that some days of the week are off. Those are easy, recovery days, offering you the chance to truly rest up for the upcoming hard workouts or races. These days are off to prevent you from slavishly following each day to the minute and not realizing that you are becoming overtrained or stale.

Remember that these are just samples based on the sacrosanct principle of hard/easy training. You can modify the days to suit your ability, current fitness level, and goals, but you must follow the pattern, which alternates between high-intensity work and low-intensity recovery.

5K Training Program To start the 5K training program (table 10.5), you should have a score of average to good or excellent on the $\dot{V}O_2$max test on page 127. If you have completed the first six weeks of the level 2 training program, you may use this program to continue your 5K training and train for better times.

In the 5K training program, all workouts except the easy, recovery jog and the long runs require 10 minutes of easy jogging at 50 to 60 percent MHR to warm up and 5 minutes of the same to cool down. These minutes are counted toward the weekly totals.

The objective of this training program is to prepare you to run the first kilometer of the race at 80 to 85 percent MHR and the second and third miles at 85 to 90 percent MHR up to 95 to 100 percent at the end of the race. This is a 14-week training program that ideally would continue the six weeks of formal heart rate training that started in level 1. You may have done much more than that, but it should have been comparable to the intensity of level 1. If you have been training harder and racing already, level 3 will help you peak for a shot at a nice new PR.

Each type of workout in the program develops a characteristic of strong running. The easy efforts help you build and maintain endurance and recover after races or hard workouts. The moderate-effort workouts improve aerobic capacity and develop your stamina. The very easy effort, indicated by the letter F on table 10.5, provides maximum recovery and tapering before a race or a really hard workout. The fast efforts develop economy. The very fast efforts develop speed.

For the long runs, indicated by the letter B on table 10.5, start slowly and let your heart rate increase as you warm into the run and slightly pick up the pace. Let effort climb to 75 percent MHR as you fatigue over the latter part of the long run.

For the uphill efforts, indicated by the letter H on table 10.5, run uphill until you reach your target heart rate zone; then recover by jogging downhill and at the bottom until your heart rate drops below 60 percent MHR. Perform the specified number of repeats.

The fast-effort interval workouts, indicated by the letter I on table 10.5, develop economy and speed. Be sure to pace yourself to reach your target heart rate zone over the last half of the interval. Do not exceed the upper limit before the end of the repeat.

10K Training Program   To start the 10K training program (table 10.6), you should have a score of average to good or excellent on the $\dot{V}O_2$max test on page 127. Or you can use this as a continuation of the level 2 training program from page 135 through week 10.

In the 10K training program, all workouts are designed around time. Therefore the distance covered will vary for each runner. Ten to 15 minutes of warm-up jogging at 50 to 60 percent MHR and 10 minutes of the same to cool down are counted toward the weekly totals. On off days, take the day off for complete rest, or if you need the minutes to reach your weekly goal, go for an easy recovery jog at 60 to 65 percent MHR. This is a 10-week training program.

Each type of workout in the program develops a characteristic of strong running. The easy efforts help you build and maintain endurance and recover after races or hard workouts. The moderate-effort workouts improve aerobic capacity and develop your stamina. The very easy effort, indicated by the letter F on table 10.5, provides maximum recovery and tapering before a race or a really hard workout. The fast efforts develop economy. The very fast efforts develop speed.

TABLE 10.5 Level 3: 5K Running Training Program

Week	Phase	Minutes per week	Days per week	Daily workout*						
				Mon.	Tues.	Wed.	Thurs.	Fri.	Sat.	Sun.
1	III	210:00	5	Off	I	45:00 A	25:00 E	Off	20:00 C	70:00 B
2	III	>150:00	5	Off	6 H	60:00 A	8 × 1:45 K	Off	30:00 F	5K race
3	III	200:00	5	45:00 A	I	Off	40:00 A	4 × D	Off	60:00 B
4	III	>150:00	5	6 × 3:30 G	Off	10 × 1:45 K	55:00 A	Off	25:00 F	5K race
5	III	190:00	5	40:00 A	8 H	Off	35:00 A	I	Off	5 × 3:30 G
6	III	>150:00	5	8 × 3:30 G	Off	4 × D	50:00 A	Off	20:00 F	5K race
7	III	180:00	5	35:00 A	12 × 1:45 K	Off	30:00 A	I	Off	48:00 B
8	III	>150:00	5	3 × D	Off	5 × 3:30 G	45:00 A	Off	20:00 F	5K race
9	IV	175:00	5	30:00 A	8 × 1:15 J	Off	30:00 A	12 × 1:45 K	Off	40:00 B
10	IV	>140:00	5	6 × 0:10 L	Off	3 × D	40:00 A	Off	20:00 F	5K race
11	IV	170:00	5	25:00 A	10 × 1:15 J	Off	35:00 A	10 × 1:45 K	Off	35:00 B
12	IV	140:00	5	I	Off	8 × 0:10 L	30:00 A	Off	15:00 F	5K race
13	IV	165:00	5	20:00 A	12 × 1:15 J	Off	35:00 A	8 × 1:45 K	Off	30:00 B
14	IV	130:00	5	10 × 0:10 L	Off	25:00 A	6 × 1:15 J	Off	15:00 F	5K race

*These are the times you should be working within your target heart rate zones. To reach the total minutes per week, include enough time to warm up and cool down.

KEY:

A: Easy effort at 65–70% MHR
B: Long run at 60–75% MHR
C: Moderate effort, steady pace at 75–80% MHR
D: Number of 7:00 repeats at 80–85% MHR with recovery intervals of slow jogging until heart rate drops below 65% MHR
E: Moderate-effort tempo running at anaerobic threshold (AT), 80–85% MHR
F: Very easy effort at 60–65% MHR
G: Fast-effort intervals at 85–90% MHR
H: Fast uphill effort at 85–90% MHR
I: Fast-effort intervals at 85–95% MHR
      1 × 7:00 at 80–85% with recovery jog to 70%
      2 × 3:30 at 85–90% with recovery jog to 65%
      4 × 1:45 at 90–95% with recovery jog to 60%
J: Very fast-effort intervals at 90–95% MHR with recovery jog until heart rate drops below 60% plus another 30 seconds of walking
K: Very fast-effort intervals at 90–95% MHR with recovery jog until heart rate drops below 60%
L: Power uphill intervals at 95–100% MHR with recovery walk or jog of 2 minutes

TABLE 10.6 Level 3: 10K Running Training Program

Week	Phase	Minutes per week	Days per week	Daily workout*						
				Mon.	Tues.	Wed.	Thurs.	Fri.	Sat.	Sun.
1	II	250:00	5	Off	50:00 A	35:00 A	30:00 E	Off	45:00 A	90:00 B
2	III	>175:00	6	45:00 A	I	45:00 A	8 × 1:45 K	Off	30:00 F	10K race
3	II	240:00	6	Off	35:00 C	45:00 A	30:00 A	25:00 E	20:00 A	85:00 B
4	III	>165:00	6	45:00 A	8 × 1:15 J	50:00 A	6 × 3:30 G	Off	25:00 F	10K race
5	II	230:00	6	Off	30:00 C	45:00 A	35:00 A	20:00 E	20:00 A	80:00 B
6	III	>155:00	6	35:00 A	10 × 1:45 K	45:00 A	6 × 1:15 J	Off	20:00 F	10K race
7	IV	180:00	5	Off	8 × 1:15 J	35:00 A	12 × 1:45 K	Off	25:00 F	70:00 B
8	IV	>155:00	5	Off	6 × 0:10 L	30:00 A	6 H	Off	20:00 F	10K race
9	III	215:00	6	30:00 A	20:00 E	40:00 A	I	25:00 A	Off	65:00 B
10	III	170:00	5	Off	8 H	30:00 A	6 × 3:30 G	Off	25:00 F	60:00 B
11	IV	>155:00	5	8 × 0:10 L	30:00 A	Off	2 × D	Off	20:00 F	10K race
12	IV	175:00	5	Off	10 × 1:45 K	30:00 A	Off	I	25:00 F	55:00 B
13	IV	155:00	5	10 H	Off	35:00 A	9 × 1:15 J	Off	25:00 F	50:00 B
14	IV	>135:00	5	Off	8 × 1:45 K	Off	6 × 1:15 J	25:00 A	15:00 F	10K race

*These are the times you should be working within your target heart rate zones. To reach the total minutes per week, include enough time to warm up and cool down.

KEY:

A: Easy effort at 65–70% MHR
B: Long run at 60–75% MHR
C: Moderate effort, steady pace at 75–80% MHR
D: Number of 7:00 repeats at 80–85% MHR with recovery intervals of slow jogging until heart rate drops below 65% MHR
E: Moderate effort, tempo running at anaerobic threshold (AT), 80–85% MHR
F: Very easy effort at 60–65% MHR
G: Fast-effort intervals at 85–90% MHR
H: Fast uphill effort at 85–90% MHR
I: Fast-effort intervals at 85–95% MHR
    1 × 7:00 at 80–85% with recovery jog to 70%
    2 × 3:30 at 85–90% with recovery jog to 65%
    4 × 1:45 at 90–95% with recovery jog to 60%
J: Very fast-effort intervals at 90–95% MHR with recovery jog until heart rate drops below 60% plus another 30 seconds of walking
K: Very fast-effort intervals at 90–95% MHR with recovery jog until heart rate drops below 60%
L: Power uphill intervals at 95–100% MHR with recovery walk or jog of 2 minutes

For the long runs, indicated by the letter B on table 10.6, start slowly and let your heart rate increase as you warm into the run and slightly pick up the pace. Let your effort climb to 75 percent MHR as you fatigue over the latter part of the long run.

For the uphill efforts, indicated by the letter H on table 10.6, run uphill until you reach your target heart rate zone; then recover by jogging downhill and at the bottom until your heart rate drops below 60 percent MHR. Perform the specified number of repeats.

The fast-effort interval workouts, indicated by the letter I on table 10.6, develop economy and speed. Be sure to pace yourself to reach your target heart rate zone over the last half of the interval. Do not exceed the upper limit before the end of the repeat.

Half Marathon Training Program The half marathon training program (table 10.7) may be used by runners who have completed level 2 through week 16 and want to train harder for a faster time. If you have a score of average to good or excellent on the $\dot{V}O_2$max test on page 127 and have adequately built your endurance, you can prepare for a 13.1-mile race using this program.

Each type of workout in the program develops a characteristic of strong running. The easy efforts help you build and maintain endurance and recover after races or hard workouts. The moderate-effort workouts improve aerobic capacity and develop your stamina. The very easy effort, indicated by the letter F on table 10.7, provides maximum recovery and tapering before a race or a really hard workout. The fast efforts develop economy. The very fast efforts develop speed.

For the long runs, indicated by the letter B on table 10.7, start slowly and let your heart rate increase as you warm into the run and slightly pick up the pace. Let effort climb to 75 percent MHR as you fatigue over the latter part of the long run.

For the uphill efforts, indicated by the letter H on table 10.7, run uphill until you reach your target heart rate zone; then recover by jogging downhill and at the bottom until your heart rate drops below 60 percent MHR. Perform the specified number of repeats.

The fast-effort interval workouts, indicated by the letter I on table 10.7, develop economy and speed. Be sure to pace yourself to reach your target heart rate zone over the last half of the interval. Do not exceed the upper limit before the end of the repeat.

Marathon Training Program This 11-week program (table 10.8) is for runners who have finished a half marathon (see level 2) or who want to run their next marathon faster.

Each type of workout in the program develops a characteristic of strong running. The easy efforts help you build and maintain endurance and recover after races or hard workouts. The moderate-effort workouts improve aerobic capacity and develop your stamina. The very easy effort, indicated by the letter F on table 10.8, provide maximum recovery and tapering before a race or a really hard workout.

For the long runs, indicated by the letter B on table 10.8, start slowly and let your heart rate increase as you warm into the run and slightly pick up the pace. Let effort climb to 75 percent MHR as you fatigue over the latter part of the long run.

TABLE 10.7 Level 3: Half Marathon Training Program										
Week	Phase	Minutes per week	Days per week	Daily workout*						
				Mon.	Tues.	Wed.	Thurs.	Fri.	Sat.	Sun.
1	I	190:00	5	25:00 A	Off	40:00 A	30:00 A	Off	35:00 A	60:00 B
2	II	260:00	5	Off	35:00 A	40:00 C	Off	20:00 E	60:00 A	105:00 B
3	III	225:00	5	Off	8 × 1:45 K	40:00 A	4 H	60:00 A	Off	90:00 B
4	II	300:00	6	35:00 C	30:00 A	45:00 A	Off	40:00 C	20:00 F	130:00 B
5	III	250:00	5	Off	10 × 1:45 K	55:00 A	Off	6 H	40:00 A	100:00 B
6	II	350:00	6	30:00 A	6 × D	25:00 A	75:00 C	Off	45:00 F	150:00 B
7	III	275:00	6	25:00 A	I	Off	45:00 A	12 × 1:15 J	25:00 F	130:00 B
8	III	250:00	6	Off	8 × 3:30 G	50:00 A	40:00 A	75:00 C	30:00 A	110:00 B
9	II	200:00	5	Off	20:00 E	30:00 A	60:00 C	Off	30:00 A	60:00 F
10	II	>155:00	7	35:00 A	30:00 A	3 × D	20:00 A	30:00 A	20:00 F	Half marathon

*These are the times you should be working within your target heart rate zones. To reach the total minutes per week, include enough time to warm up and cool down.

KEY:

A: Easy effort at 65–70% MHR
B: Long run at 60–75% MHR
C: Moderate effort, steady pace at 75–80% MHR
D: Number of 7:00 repeats at 80–85% MHR with recovery intervals of slow jogging until heart rate drops below 65% MHR
E: Moderate effort, tempo running at anaerobic threshold (AT), 80–85% MHR
F: Very easy effort at 60–65% MHR
G: Fast-effort intervals at 85–90% MHR
H: Fast uphill effort at 85–90% MHR
I: Fast-effort intervals at 85–95% MHR
　　　1 × 7:00 at 80–85% with recovery jog to 70%
　　　2 × 3:30 at 85–90% with recovery jog to 65%
　　　4 × 1:45 at 90–95% with recovery jog to 60%
J: Very fast-effort intervals at 90–95% MHR with recovery jog until heart rate drops below 60% plus another 30 seconds of walking
K: Very fast-effort intervals at 90–95% MHR with recovery jog until heart rate drops below 60%

TABLE 10.8 Level 3: Marathon Training Program

Week	Phase	Minutes per week	Days per week	Daily workout*						
				Mon.	Tues.	Wed.	Thurs.	Fri.	Sat.	Sun.
1	I	190:00	5	25:00 A	35:00 A	Off	35:00 A	30:00 A	Off	55:00 A
2	I	320:00	7	40:00 A	25:00 C	45:00 A	30:00 A	30:00 C	35:00 A	115:00 B
3	II	375:00	5	Off	45:00 C	75:00 A	Off	55:00 C	65:00 F	135:00 B
4	II	480:00	7	50:00 A	35:00 C	65:00 A	50:00 A	65:00 C	60:00 F	160:00 B
5	III	300:00	6	45:00 A	25:00 E	Off	55:00 A	5 × D	35:00 F	100:00 B
6	II	520:00	7	45:00 A	6 × D	80:00 A	65:00 A	70:00 C	60:00 F	170:00 B
7	III	315:00	6	Off	45:00 A	30:00 E	60:00 A	6 × D	25:00 F	110:00 B
8	II	560:00	7	45:00 A	55:00 C	75:00 A	75:00 C	65:00 A	50:00 F	180:00 B
9	III	325:00	6	Off	45:00 A	35:00 E	60:00 A	7 × D	25:00 F	120:00 B
10	II	260:00	6	40:00 C	45:00 C	30:00 A	Off	40:00 C	30:00 F	75:00 A
11	II	> 170:00	7	40:00 A	3 × D	25:00 A	40:00 C	25:00 A	15:00 A	Marathon

*These are the times you should be working within your target heart rate zones. To reach the total minutes per week, include enough time to warm up and cool down.

KEY:

A: Easy effort at 65–70% MHR
B: Long run at 60–75% MHR
C: Moderate effort, steady pace at 75–80% MHR
D: Number of 7:00 repeats at 80–85% MHR with recovery intervals of slow jogging until heart rate drops below 65% MHR
E: Moderate effort, tempo running at anaerobic threshold (AT), 80–85% MHR
F: Very easy effort at 60–65% MHR

Continuing Your Training

These training programs were designed to help you appreciate how to individualize your training. They are examples of smart, not just hard, work. If you seek improvement, keep this revelation in mind: Once you have experienced what drop-dead, all-out exhaustion feels like at 100-percent effort, it never gets any harder. Every all-out, 100-percent effort after that will feel the same—painful, agonizing breathlessness. The good news is that your other training zones also will feel the same—some easy, some medium, some hard. So what do you do if you can't train harder but want to get better? Simple—you run more. Go back and add more minutes to these training programs. As you run more, you will get stronger. The stronger you get, the faster you will run.

CHAPTER 11

Cycling

Cycling, at its highest levels, tests the limits of endurance like few other activities do. Few sports require you to perform at race pace for multiple days in a row. The most obvious cycling challenge is the Tour de France, which is made up of 21 days of racing over 23 days—but not too many of us are likely to qualify for this ride. These multiday races present formidable challenges in many areas including aerobic fitness, anaerobic fitness, nutrition, and perhaps most important, recovery.

Of course, this level of performance is a long way from our starting point, which is a basic program to build cardiorespiratory fitness. Eight weeks of this is followed by another eight weeks of working in areas of anaerobic fitness and power development. We conclude with a 12-week century training program that has as a starting requirement the capacity to do a 90-minute ride (in other words, you have completed the equivalent of the level 1 program).

Because of the nature of the sport, people often ride their bikes longer than they would run or swim. With the exception of time trials and criteriums, bike races usually require riders to be in the saddle for several hours, versus only minutes for activities such as swimming or rowing, or 30 to 60 minutes for 5K and 10K running races.

With that said, the physiology of competitive cycling requires a huge engine (large $\dot{V}O_2max$) and therefore a particular combination of body weight and training. For this reason, the hours spent bike training are long and, if indoors, can be boring. However, the rewards can come quickly, because spending several hours working out at a time reaps good payback fairly quickly in terms of both fitness and weight loss.

Given the variety of cycling abilities and the fact that there are more than five rating categories in competitive cycling, creating a generic program that will benefit all cyclists is difficult. Our goal is not to make you world class, although we can if you wish. Rather, our goal is to guide you through a starting program, either indoors or outdoors, and then help you systematically

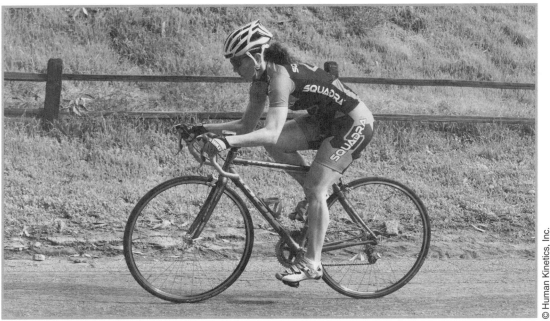

© Human Kinetics, Inc.

Cycling training may be done indoors or outdoors. After building a base of endurance, cycling training moves into increasing anaerobic capacity and power.

build on your fitness by developing your anaerobic and power abilities. You will do this using heart rate training and working through the various phases in the four-phase training methodology.

The training program for a beginner rider lasts eight weeks and focuses primarily on cardiorespiratory fitness. Next comes the higher-intensity, or intermediate, fitness level, in which we increase the intensity and speed. This program also is eight weeks long. From here you can continue to repeat level 2 because your heart rate will naturally adapt and allow you to adjust your intensity. What you'll notice is that your work rate is steadily increasing while your heart rate is staying the same, another good reason to make sure you keep good records of workouts including heart rates and workloads. The programs are progressive and are based on our four-phase training philosophy. The four phases are referred to as zones 1 through 4 in the program.

As with many endurance sports, the option to exercise indoors exists in cycling. Often, riding indoors gives greater control over intensity and conditions. For our program we are assuming that you will ride both indoors and outdoors and therefore have a fairly high degree of variability in heart rate given hills, wind, and other environmental variables. In this program, heart rate prescriptions are often spread across two heart rate training zones because this is a more typical experience, especially when cycling outdoors. (Actually, variability is spread across four training zones, but you can avoid the upper zones by going easier on hills.)

The bonus program, the century training program, is more of a seasonal, or ultimate, goal that you can work toward when you have the time. Given the popularity of century rides these days, we decided it would be a nice addition. Just remember that the century ride program has a minimum requirement of being able to ride for 90 minutes continuously.

One last consideration: Cycling, like rowing and swimming, is highly technical. Believe it or not, there is correct form in bike riding that includes pedaling cadence, efficiency, body position, and other factors. These are important components in any program designed to improve cycling performance, and you should also consider drills designed to improve these aspects of riding. We concentrate only on the progressions and workouts needed to develop the fitness component of cycling. Table 11.1 highlights the four training phases.

TABLE 11.1 Cycling Training Phases

Training phase	Percent MHR
Phase I: Endurance (EZ)	60–75%
Phase II: Stamina (MO)	75–85%
Phase III: Economy (FA)	85–95%
Phase IV: Speed (VF)	95–100%

Classifying Your Current Fitness Level

Use this simple bike test adapted from Anderson (1995) to classify your current fitness. You will need a bike that can measure watts. Start at 35 watts and increase the wattage by 35 watts every 2 minutes until you can no longer maintain the power output.

Table 11.2 lists approximate maximum oxygen consumption in liters per minute for the wattage of the work output. Simply multiply this by 1,000 to get milliliters, and then divide by your body mass in kilograms. This will give you your $\dot{V}O_2max$ in ml/kg/min. Compare your result to table 11.3 if you are male or table 11.4 if you are female.

For example, let's consider the case of a 35-year-old male who weighs 70 kilograms and reaches 315 watts on the test. His $\dot{V}O_2max$ would be

$$3.84 \times 1,000 = 3,840 / 70 = 54.8 \text{ ml/kg/min}$$

According to table 11.3, he would be classified as average. His starting point for fitness training would be level 2.

Test adapted from Anderson, L.B., 1995, A maximal exercise protocol to predict maximal oxygen uptake, *Scandinavian Journal of Medicine and Science in Sports*, pages 143–146.

TABLE 11.2 $\dot{V}O_2$max in Liters per Minute per Wattage

Wattage	$\dot{V}O_2$max (liters/minute)
35	0.56
70	0.97
105	1.38
140	1.79
175	2.20
210	2.61
245	3.02
280	3.43
315	3.84
350	4.25
385	4.66
420	5.07
455	5.48
490	5.80
525	6.30

TABLE 11.3 Fitness Classifications Based on $\dot{V}O_2$max Results: Male Athletes

Age	Poor	Fair	Average	Good	Excellent
15–19	≤52	53–57	58–65	66–69	≥70
20–29	≤52	53–59	60–69	70–77	≥78
30–39	≤47	48–53	54–62	63–71	≥72
40–49	≤39	40–43	44–55	56–63	≥64
50–59	≤31	32–37	38–51	52–57	≥58
60–69	≤22	23–30	31–42	43–54	≥55
	Level 1		Level 2		Level 3

Note: Classifications reflect conditioning status for endurance athletes. Data for nonathletes would be much lower.

TABLE 11.4	Fitness Classifications Based on $\dot{V}O_2$max Results: Female Athletes				
Age	Poor	Fair	Average	Good	Excellent
15–19	≤48	49–54	55–61	62–67	≥68
20–29	≤49	50–54	55–62	63–71	≥72
30–39	≤39	40–49	50–55	56–64	≥65
40–49	≤28	29–40	41–48	49–59	≥60
50–59	≤19	20–28	29–40	41–50	≥51
60–69	≤7	8–14	15–25	26–41	≥42
	Level 1		Level 2		Level 3

Note: Classifications reflect conditioning status for endurance athletes. Data for nonathletes would be much lower.

Determining Your Cycling Training Zones

In chapter 2, we provided a simple protocol for determining your maximum heart rate (MHR). Use that protocol here to get your maximum heart rate number and then calculate your various heart rate zones—60 to 75 percent, 75 to 80 percent, and so on. This will allow you to determine your training zones.

Determining Your Cycling Maximum Heart Rate

1. Find a strong climb that is 600 to 1,000 meters long. Ideally, there will be a loop where you can get a 2- to 3-mile (3.2 to 4.8 km) recovery.
2. Bike for a 5- to 8-mile (8 to 13 km) warm-up.
3. After the warm-up, climb the hill as fast as you can. During the climb, get out of the saddle for the last 70 to 100 meters and push as hard as you can.
4. Bike a 2- to 3-mile (3.2 to 4.8 km) recovery and repeat the climb.
5. Bike a 2- to 3-mile (3.2 to 4.8 km) recovery and repeat the climb again. Your heart rate at the end of this third trial should be a good indicator of your maximum heart rate.

Choosing a Training Program

Knowing which program to start with is usually the initial question. Be conservative when choosing a beginning program. Often, people look at a program and think, "I can do that easily enough," but when faced with the increase in volume, they have difficulty or end up injured. Use this guideline: It's not what you think you *can* do; it's what you have normally been doing. If you regularly exercise three or four times a week, you might be able to jump to level 2 right away. If not, then start at level 1. Also, keep in mind that cycling is very different from other forms of exercise. If cycling hasn't been part of your exercise repertoire, start at level 1.

Each program has an objective. However, unlike some activities, such as running, the nature of cycling allows all programs to contain a mix of intensities. In cycling, the risk of injury is a little lower, and you can recover somewhat more easily on a bike and still keep moving. You will notice greater variety particularly in level 2 when the objectives of the program extend beyond basic cardiorespiratory fitness.

Level 1

The level 1 program (table 11.5) is a basic introductory program to get you over the initial saddle sores and to help you develop a little fitness along the way. It is conservative in its progression for the first four weeks and then ramps up a bit in week 5 with the addition of some higher-intensity work, which you will be ready for at that time.

TABLE 11.5 Level 1 Cycling Training Program: Endurance and Stamina

Week	Mon.	Tues.	Wed.	Thurs.	Fri.	Sat.	Sun.
1	Off	30:00 EZ	Off	30:00 EZ	30:00 EZ	Off	30:00 EZ
2	Off	45:00 EZ	Off	45:00 EZ	45:00 EZ	Off	45:00 EZ
3	Off	60:00 EZ	Off	60:00 EZ	60:00 EZ	Off	60:00 EZ
4	Off	75:00 EZ	Off	75:00 EZ	75:00 EZ	Off	75:00 EZ
5	Off	90:00 EZ-MO	Off	90:00 EZ-MO	Off	60:00 EZ-MO	90:00 EZ-MO
6	Off	90:00 EZ-MO	60:00 EZ-MO	60:00 EZ-MO	Off	90:00 EZ-MO	90:00 EZ-MO
7	Off	90:00 EZ-MO	60:00 EZ-MO	60:00 EZ-MO	Off	60:00 EZ-MO	90:00 EZ-MO
8	Off	60:00 EZ-MO	Off	60:00 EZ-MO	Off	Off	25 mi. (40 km)

KEY:

EZ: Endurance training at 60–75% MHR
MO: Stamina training at 75–80% MHR

Level 2

Successful completion of the level 1 program will result in a sound and safe cardiorespiratory base. The progression to level 2 consists primarily of increases in duration with slight increases in intensity toward the latter weeks. Level 2, in addition to further increases in intensity, includes some introductory-level intervals and also some significant increases in time spent in the saddle. Table 11.6 details the training program, and table 11.7 lists the interval sessions. You will notice a greater variety in the type of workouts in this program, even though there is a defined goal of economy and speed endurance. This variety of workouts further develops your fitness and performance levels. The additional programs in table 11.8 and table 11.9 that focus on the triathlon sprint cycling distances of 14 miles (22.5 km) and 28 miles (45 km) focus more on intensity than duration.

TABLE 11.6 Level 2 Cycling Training Program: Economy and Speed Endurance

Week	Mon.	Tues.	Wed.	Thurs.	Fri.	Sat.	Sun.
9	Off	90:00 EZ-MO	Off	90:00 EZ-MO	Off	60:00 EZ-MO	90:00–120:00 EZ-MO
10	Off	90:00 EZ-MO	60:00 A1	90:00 EZ-MO	Off	90:00 EZ-MO	90:00–150:00 EZ-MO
11	Off	90:00 EZ-MO	75:00 EZ-MO	75:00 EZ-MO	Off	60:00 A1	90:00–150:00 EZ-MO
12	Off	90:00 EZ-MO	Off	90:00 EZ-MO	Off	60:00 A1	90:00–120:00 EZ-MO
13	Off	90:00 EZ-MO	75:00 A2	90:00 EZ-MO	Off	60:00 A1	90:00–150:00 EZ-MO
14	Off	90:00 EZ-MO	75:00 A2 15:00 EZ	75:00 EZ-MO	Off	60:00 A1 15:00 EZ	90:00–150:00 EZ-MO
15	Off	60:00 EZ-MO	75:00 A2 15:00 EZ	60:00 EZ-MO	Off	60:00 A1 15:00 EZ	90:00–150:00 EZ-MO
16	Off	60:00 EZ-MO	75:00 A2 15:00 EZ	60:00 EZ-MO	Off	Off	90:00–150:00 EZ-MO

KEY:

EZ: Endurance training at 60–75% MHR
MO: Stamina training at 75–80% MHR
A1: Intervals; see table 11.7.
A2: Intervals; see table 11.7.

TABLE 11.7 Level 2 Cycling Training Program: A1 and A2 Intervals*

A1 intervals		A2 intervals	
Time	Percent MHR	Time	Percent MHR
0:00–6:00	<60%	0:00–6:00	<60%
6:00–12:00	65–70%	6:00–12:00	65–70%
12:00–18:00	80–90%	12:00–18:00	80–90%
18:00–24:00	65–70%	18:00–24:00	65–70%
24:00–30:00	80–90%	24:00–30:00	80–90%
30:00–36:00	65–70%	30:00–36:00	65–70%
36:00–38:00	>90%	36:00–42:00	>90%
38:00–44:00	65–70%	42:00–48:00	65–70%
44:00–46:00	80–90%	48:00–54:00	80–90%
46:00–52:00	65–70%	54:00–60:00	65–70%
52:00–54:00	>90%	60:00–66:00	>90%
54:00–60:00	<60%	66:00–75:00	<60%

*All intervals are performed at 70–80 rpm.

TABLE 11.8 Level 2 Cycling Training Program: Four-Week Training for Sprint Triathlon Distance (12–15 mi; 19–24 km)

Week	Mon.	Tues.	Wed.	Thurs.	Fri.	Sat.	Sun.
1	30:00 EZ	Off	30:00 EZ	Off	30:00 EZ	30:00 EZ	Off
2	45:00 EZ	Off	45:00 EZ	Off	45:00 EZ	45:00 EZ	Off
3	60:00 EZ	Off	60:00 EZ	Off	60:00 EZ	60:00 EZ	Off
4	75:00 EZ	Off	75:00 EZ	Off	75:00 EZ	75:00 EZ	Off

KEY:

EZ: heart rate zone 1

TABLE 11.9 Level 2 Cycling Training Program: Four-Week Training for Olympic Triathlon Distance (24–28 mi; 39–45 km)*

Week	Mon.	Tues.	Wed.	Thurs.	Fri.	Sat.	Sun.
1	60:00 EZ	Off	60:00 EZ	Off	60:00 EZ	Off	60:00 EZ
2	75:00 EZ	Off	75:00 EZ	Off	75:00 EZ	Off	75:00 EZ
3	90:00 EZ-MO	Off	90:00 EZ-MO	Off	Off	60:00 EZ-MO	90:00 EZ-MO
4	90:00 EZ-MO	Off	60:00 EZ-MO	60:00 EZ-MO	Off	90:00 EZ-MO	90:00 EZ-MO

*This program assumes an ability to complete the sprint triathlon training program shown in table 11.8.

KEY:

EZ: heart rate zone 1
MO: heart rate zone 2

150 •

Level 3

The level 3 training program (table 11.10) takes something of a reversal in approach with a larger amount of time given back to easy and moderate work, but again, there is a significant increase in the amount of time spent in the saddle. At this stage you'll appreciate the value of a pair of nicely padded shorts.

	TABLE 11.10 Level 3 Cycling Training Program: 12-Week Training for Half Ironman Distance* (56 mi; 90 km)						
Week	**Mon.**	**Tues.**	**Wed.**	**Thurs.**	**Fri.**	**Sat.**	**Sun.**
1	Off	60:00 EZ-MO	Off	60:00 EZ-MO	Off	60:00 EZ-MO	60:00–90:00 EZ-MO
2	Off	75:00 EZ-MO	Off	75:00 EZ-MO	Off	75:00 EZ-MO	75:00–120:00 EZ-MO
3	Off	90:00 EZ-MO	Off	75:00 EZ-MO	Off	60:00 A1	90:00–120:00 EZ-MO
4	Off	90:00 EZ-MO	Off	90:00 EZ-MO	Off	60:00 A1	90:00–120:00 EZ-MO
5	Off	60:00 EZ-MO	75:00 A2	Off	Off	60:00 A1	120:00–150:00 EZ-MO
6	Off	60:00 EZ-MO	75:00 A2 15:00 EZ	75:00 EZ-MO	Off	Off	120:00–150:00 EZ-MO
7	Off	60:00 EZ-MO	75:00 A2 15:00 EZ	60:00 EZ-MO	Off	Off	120:00–150:00 EZ-MO
8	Off	60:00 EZ-MO	75:00 A2 15:00 EZ	60:00 EZ-MO	Off	Off	120:00–150:00 EZ-MO
9	Off	75:00 EZ-MO	75:00 A2 15:00 EZ	Off	Off	150:00 EZ	150:00 EZ
10	Off	75:00 EZ-MO	75:00 A2 15:00 EZ	Off	Off	150:00 EZ	180:00 EZ
11	Off	90:00 EZ-MO	75:00 A2 15:00 EZ	Off	Off	150:00 EZ	180:00 EZ
12	Off	75:00 EZ-MO	45:00 EZ	Off	Off	56 mi. (90 km)	Off

*This program assumes the completion of level 1 training.

KEY:

EZ: heart rate zone 1
MO: heart rate zone 2

Bonus Century Training Program

The bonus century ride program contains a large increase over level 3 in time spent in the saddle. Table 11.11 details the program, and table 11.12 lists the interval sessions. You may have noted that there are longer distances for cycling, such as the 112 miles (180 km) for the Ironman. In reality, the distance of 100 miles (161 km) versus 112 miles (180), which is the full Ironman distance, is not that great at this level of participation. Anyone who successfully completes the century training program will not have any additional challenge in going the 112-mile (180 km) distance. The goal here

TABLE 11.11 Century Ride Training Program

Week	Mon.	Tues.	Wed.	Thurs.	Fri.	Sat.	Sun.
1	Off	90:00 EZ-MO	1:00:00 IT1	1:30:00 EZ-MO	Off	2:00:00 EZ-MO	1:30:00 EZ
2	Off	90:00 EZ-MO	1:00:00 IT1	1:30:00 EZ-MO	Off	2:00:00 EZ-MO	1:30:00 EZ
3	Off	90:00 EZ-MO	1:15:00 IT2	1:30:00 EZ-MO	Off	2:30:00 EZ-MO	1:00:00 EZ
4	Off	1:00:00 EZ	1:15:00 IT2	1:30:00 EZ-MO	Off	3:00:00 EZ-MO	1:30:00 EZ
5	2:00:00 IT3	Off	1:30:00 EZ-MO	2:30:00 EZ-MO	Off	4:00:00 EZ-MO	Off
6	2:00:00 IT3	Off	1:30:00 IT4	Off	2:00:00 EZ-MO	4:30:00 EZ-MO	2:00:00 EZ-MO
7	Off	Off	2:00:00 IT3	2:30:00 EZ-MO	Off	5:00:00 EZ-MO	Off
8	2:00:00 IT3	1:00:00 EZ-MO	Off	1:30:00 IT4	Off	5:30:00 EZ-MO	Off
9	Off	1:30:00 EZ-MO	Off	2:30:00 EZ-MO	1:30:00 EZ-MO	6:00:00 EZ-MO	Off
10	Off	3:00:00 EZ-MO	3:00:00 EZ-MO	1:30:00 IT4	Off	6:00:00 EZ-MO	Off
11	Off	3:00:00 EZ-MO	2:00:00 EZ-MO	Off	Off	2:00:00 EZ-MO	2:00:00 EZ-MO
12	2:00:00 IT3	Off	Off	1:30:00 EZ-MO	Off	Off	Century

KEY:

EZ: Endurance training at 60–75% MHR
MO: Stamina training at 75–80% MHR
IT1: Intervals; see table 11.12.
IT2: Intervals; see table 11.12.
IT3: Intervals; see table 11.12.
IT4: Intervals; see table 11.12.

TABLE 11.12	Interval Training Sessions for Century Training Program		
Interval 1*	**Interval 2**	**Interval 3**	**Interval 4**
20:00 EZ	20:00 EZ	30:00 EZ	20:00 EZ
5:00 FA-VF	5:00 FA-VF	10:00 MO	5:00 FA-VF
10:00 EZ	10:00 EZ	40:00 FA-VF	10:00 EZ
5:00 FA-VF	5:00 FA-VF	40:00 EZ	5:00 FA-VF
20:00 EZ	10:00 EZ		10:00 EZ
	5:00 FA-VF		5:00 FA-VF
	20:00 EZ		10:00 EZ
			5:00 FA-VF
			20:00 EZ

*For interval 1 and interval 2, ideally 5:00 FA should be short climbs. For interval 3, ideally the 40:00 FA-VF is a long climb.

KEY:

EZ: Endurance training at 60–75% MHR
MO: Stamina training at 75–80% MHR
FA: Economy training at 80–90% MHR
VF: Speed training at 90–100% MHR

is to allow you to complete the 100-mile ride in six to seven hours or with an average speed of 14 to 16 miles per hour (22.5 to 25.7 km/h). Please note that the rest days include the option of complete rest or a swim session, but no running or biking.

Continuing Your Training

Getting fit is the hard part. Staying fit is usually a little easier and requires less work, although typically it involves a bit more intensity. Fitness can be maintained by dropping from five or six sessions per week back to three or four sessions per week as long as you maintain a higher overall intensity.

As with swimming, cycling fitness tends to limit itself to the act of cycling. Although you will develop great cardiorespiratory fitness, it will have little transferability to any other activity. Be careful if you decide to jump off your bike and go for a run because this transition requires a little practice. On the plus side, cycling is one of a very few activities that allows you to exercise for hours and not beat your joints with pounding. For that reason, it is a beneficial and enjoyable exercise option for those who want to exercise longer.

CHAPTER 12

Swimming

Of all the endurance activities that we cover in this book, swimming has the potential to create the most challenges. Swimming is a complex activity requiring a lot of skill, and as such results in varied levels of exertion. As many of us find out, increased effort in the water doesn't always result in increased speed. This is because of the skill and technique swimming requires. Unlike running, swimming does not come naturally; we have to learn it. For that reason, swim training involves more drills and skill activities than any of the other popular endurance sports. Add to that the number of strokes that exist and you end up with a very challenging situation. Getting fitter in the water doesn't always mean getting faster because this also depends on skill level. On the other hand, we've all seen chubby swimmers who glide through the water with relative ease.

Another important difference between swimming and other activities is that breathing is highly regulated. You can breathe only at certain times, at a particular phase in the stroke and when the face is out of the water. Breathing is particularly challenging because poor breathing mechanics artificially increase stress levels, thereby affecting heart rate in a way not related to the intensity of the exercise.

Before we get into programming, we need to consider the unique physiology of swimming. Heart rate response in particular is affected by the horizontal position and the water pressure. These are some of the reasons that, for most people, maximum heart rate (MHR) is much lower in the water than on land. Only when the person has become very well trained in the water is she capable of producing close to her equivalent land-based aerobic heart rate, albeit still at about 10 bpm lower. In our experience, a person swimming at a steady state will have a heart rate that is 25 to 40 bpm lower than his heart rate during steady state exercise on land. Thus, heart rate training zones also are considerably lower in the water.

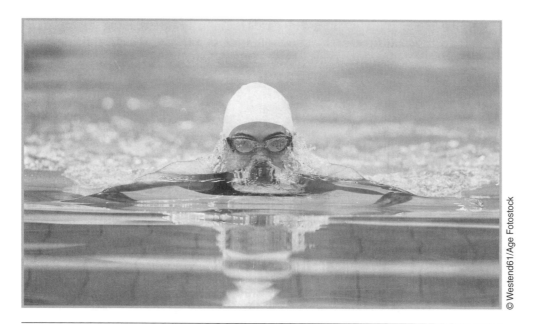

Because of the nature of the sport, swimmers usually have a lower maximum heart rate in the water than they do on land.

One final anomaly about swimming relates to the distance swimmers cover in training. Most swimming events are less than 2 minutes long, with many events lasting less than 1 minute; yet swimmers log the equivalent of marathon training hours. As physiologists, we struggle to explain this in terms of energy system adaptations. From a motor control point of view, it does make sense to learn the skill by repeating the movement over and over. But once the skill is learned, it would seem logical to focus more specifically on the energy systems required for a particular event. We kept this issue in mind when we created the swimming training programs in this chapter.

We do make some assumptions about swimming ability in the programs outlined in this chapter. We assume that you already can swim and can repeat the sets, taking whatever rest you need to move on to the next set.

Classifying Your Current Fitness Level

Fitness testing for swimming is a little more complex than fitness testing for a land-based activity such as running. Swimming is a complex skill that can be favorably affected by higher body fat levels, a factor that can negatively affect performance in land-based activities. People with relatively low cardiorespiratory fitness actually can perform quite well in swimming, particularly distance swimming. The best way to classify swimming fitness is to base it on a timed swim for a set distance. The following protocol is for a timed 500-yard (457.2 m) swim.

Perform a warm-up of 100 to 200 yards (91.4 to 182.8 m) using the freestyle stroke. Rest for 2 minutes; then swim 500 yards (457.2 m) as fast as you can. Compare your time to determine your fitness level:

Beginner: More than 11:40

Novice: 9:30 to 11:39

Expert: Less than 9:30

The classification system is based on the freestyle, or front crawl. These numbers are based on data from the U.S. Navy and don't differentiate between males and females. Swimming is one of the few sports in which female scores are fairly close to male scores. In fact, when the distances increase, the time gap narrows; many long-distance swimming records are held by females. Use this classification to guide you to the right program for you.

Determining Your Swimming Training Zones

You have two options for finding your swimming training zones: (1) Determine your initial fitness classification, or (2) determine your maximum heart rate and your heart rate at your critical swim speed. It is possible to get both maximum heart rate and fitness classification information from the 500-yard timed swim test described previously. However, we have a second option for you. If you have time, complete both tests and collect the heart rate data during both. From there you'll be able to go on and start a training program.

Programs 1 and 2 are based on heart rate and require a little homework at first. The first assignment is to calculate your maximum heart rate while swimming. The second is to calculate your heart rate at your critical swim speed, or swimming anaerobic threshold speed. From there you can calculate your swimming anaerobic threshold heart rate.

Determining Your Swimming Maximum Heart Rate

Remember, all maximum tests require a maximum effort in terms of both cardiovascular function and muscle contraction forces and velocities. Therefore, check with your doctor to make sure you are ready and capable of performing the tests and have the necessary background to proceed. Perform a 500-yard (457.2 m) warm-up at a slow to moderate pace. Then swim 100 yards as fast as you can three times with 30-second rests between sets. Record your heart rate at the end of the third 100 yards (91.4 m). This represents your maximum heart rate while swimming.

Using your maximum heart rate, calculate your training zones by applying the formula percentages associated with the various training phases. Keep in mind that most people experience maximum heart rates in the order of 10 to 20 bpm lower during swimming than they do during running or cycling. Do not be alarmed to see these lower numbers. Numerous factors account for this difference, including body position, hydrostatic pressure, cooling effect of the water temperature, and regulated breathing, among others.

Your fitness classification determines your starting program. As a general rule, progress through the fitness programs in ascending order, from level 1 to level 2 and then to level 3. If you believe you are ready to start with level 2, make sure you meet the ending requirement of the level 1 program: a continuous swim of 1,650 yards (1,509 m).

Determining Your Swimming Anaerobic Threshold

Because the level 1 program is designed to raise your level of fitness, you really don't need to determine your swimming anaerobic threshold until you are ready to progress to level 2. Before starting level 2, you need to assess your anaerobic threshold because doing so will allow you to more accurately pinpoint training phases III and IV.

The critical swim test was developed by Ginn (E. Ginn. 1993. *Critical speed and training intensities for swimming.* Australian Sports Commission.). Following a 500-yard warm-up, perform 50-meter and 400-meter swims as fast as possible. Swim the 50 meters first and rest for 3 minutes before swimming the 400 meters. Record times for both swims; then apply this formula:

Critical swim speed in meters per second (m/s) = $(D2 - D1) / (T2 - T1)$

in which D is distance and T is time in seconds. For example, let's say a swimmer swims the 50 meters in 31 seconds and the 400 meters in 5 minutes (300 seconds). The formula would look like this:

Critical swim speed in m/s = $(400 - 50) / (300 - 31) = 350 / 269 = 1.30$ m/s

This indicates a critical swim speed, or a swim speed at anaerobic threshold, of 1.30 meters per second. Now you need to translate this into heart rate. An athlete swimming 1.30 meters per second will swim one length of a 25-meter pool in 19.23 seconds. He would need to swim 500 yards (457.2 m) at 19.23 seconds per 25 meters to record the average heart rate over distance. This is his swimming AT threshold. Let's assume it comes out to be 132 bpm, or 80 percent MHR (166 bpm). These numbers provide the guidance we need to develop a longer, more focused program for level 2.

Choosing a Training Program

This chapter presents three programs that are progressive—each one is built on the previous one. We start with a basic introductory program (level 1) designed to improve cardiorespiratory fitness. The majority of this program takes place in the endurance (EZ) zone. The specific heart rates for all four training phases are shown in table 12.1. You will notice a slight difference in the zone percentage for swimming. This correction is made due to the varied HR response in the water. The level 2 and 3 programs build on this cardiorespiratory fitness while also developing anaerobic capacity and speed. Before proceeding to the next level, make sure you meet the goal of your current level. (For example, if you classify to start at level 2 make sure you

TABLE 12.1 Swimming Training Phases	
Training phase	**Percent MHR**
Phase I: Endurance (EZ)	60–75%
Phase II: Stamina (MO)	75–80%
Phase III: Economy (FA)	80–90%
Phase IV: Speed endurance (VF)	90–100%

can complete the ending requirements of level 1.) In accordance with our training phases, levels 2 and 3 build on economy and speed endurance, also called anaerobic power and speed. You can repeat any level by continuing to work at the same heart rate. What you'll notice is that your split times for the distances covered will start to drop. Keeping good records will help you track these adaptations.

Level 1

The goal of the level 1 program (table 12.2) is to build cardiorespiratory endurance by increasing the distance up to a swimmer's mile (1,650 yd or 1,509 m). By Friday of week 6, you should be able to swim 1,650 yards (1,509 m) in heart rate training zone 2 with no rest.

TABLE 12.2 Level 1 Swimming Training Program				
Week	**Days of week**	**Zone**	**Workout**	**Total distance**
1	Mon., Wed., Fri.	EZ	4 × 100 yd, 1:00 rest between reps 5 × 50 yd, 0:30 rest between reps 6 × 25 yd, 0:15 rest between reps	800 yd
2	Mon., Wed., Fri.	EZ	150 yd, 1:30 rest 4 × 100 yd, 1:00 rest between reps 5 × 50 yd, 0:30 rest between reps 6 × 25 yd, 0:15 rest between reps	950 yd
3	Mon., Wed., Fri.	EZ	2 × 300 yd, 2:00 rest between reps 4 × 150 yd, 1:30 rest between reps	1,200 yd
4	Mon., Wed., Fri.	EZ MO	2 × 600 yd, 3:00 rest between reps 4 × 200 yd, 1:30 rest between reps	2,000 yd
5	Mon., Wed., Fri.	EZ MO	1,200 yd, 3:00 rest 2 × 400 yd, 2:00 rest between reps	2,000 yd
6	Mon., Wed., Fri.	EZ MO	2 × 1,200 yd, 1:00 rest between reps 1,650 yd, no rest	2,400 yd + 1,650 yd for Friday swim

Swimmer's mile = 1,650 yards
For English-to-metric conversions, visit www.worldwidemetric.com/measurements.html.

KEY:
EZ: heart rate zone 1
MO: heart rate zone 2

Level 2

The goal of the six-week level 2 program (table 12.3) is to enhance cardiore-spiratory fitness (EZ) and begin work on stamina (MO).

In the workouts noted in table 12.3, the word *kick* means to use a kick-board for part of the workout. For example, the instruction in workout A (EZ 6 × 100 yd free with 25 yd kick) means to swim freestyle for 100 yards and then use a kickboard for 25 yards, repeating the pattern six times. When *choice* is noted, you can use any stroke. *Ladder up alternate pull* means to swim the yards noted, alternating between a regular swim and a pull swim in which you have a buoy between your legs. For example, in the Tuesday workout (workout B), you swim 25 yards, pull 50 yards, swim 75 yards, pull 100 yards, and so on up the ladder. The phrase *alternate pull* means to swim one set and then pull a buoy in the next set. HR stands for *heart rate*. For English-to-metric conversions of the distances in the workouts, visit www.worldwidemetric.com/measurements.html.

For the time trial (TT in table 12.3), warm up for 600 yards (548.6 m) at an easy pace (heart rate less than 65 percent MHR) and then swim 1,650 yards (1,509 m) and time your effort. After 1,650 yards, cool down by swimming 300 yards (274.3 m) at an easy pace (less than 65 percent MHR). Record your result.

Workout A

Total distance: 2,450 yd

Warm-up: EZ 600 yd (HR <65%)

EZ 6 × 100 yd free with 25 yd kick (total of 125 yd) (HR <75%)

EZ 5 × 100 yd: 50 yd EZ (HR <75%) followed by 50 yd fast

EZ 6 × 50 yd: 25 EZ then 25 fast

Cool-down: EZ 300 yd choice (HR <65%)

TABLE 12.3 Level 2 Swimming Training Program: Cardiorespiratory Fitness and Stamina

Week	Mon.	Tues.	Wed.	Thurs.	Fri.
1	A (2,450 yd)	B (2,600 yd)	C (2,600 yd)	D (1,900 yd)	E (3,250 yd)
2	F (2,950 yd)	B (2,600 yd)	E (3,250 yd)	D (1,900 yd)	A (2,450 yd)
3	TT (2,550 yd)	H (3,300 yd)	D (1,900 yd)	G (2,800 yd)	E (3,250 yd)
4	H (3,300 yd)	E (3,250 yd)	D (1,900 yd)	A (2,450 yd)	I (4,250 yd)
5	TT (2,550 yd)	H (3,300 yd)	D (1,900 yd)	G (2,800 yd)	E (3,250 yd)
6	H (3,300 yd)	E (3,250 yd)	D (1,900 yd)	A (2,450 yd)	I (4,025 yd)

See chapter text for descriptions of workouts A through I. For English-to-metric conversions, visit www.worldwidemetric.com/measurements.html.

KEY:

TT: Time trial

Workout B

Total distance: 2,600 yd

Warm-up: EZ 600 yd (HR <65%)

Ladder up alternate pull, no rest, EZ (25, 50, 75, 100, 125, 150, 175, 200) (HR <75%)

EZ 4 × 200 yd alternating 50 yd easy, 50 yd fast, 50 yd easy pull, 50 yd fast (HR <75%)

Cool-down: EZ 300 yd choice (HR <65%)

Workout C

Total distance: 2,600 yd

Warm-up: EZ 600 yd (HR <65%)

Pull MO 500 yd (HR <80%)

Pull 6 × 100 yd fast with 50 yd easy (HR <75%)

MO 6 × 50 yd, rest for 1:30 between sets (HR <80%)

Cool-down: EZ 300 yd choice (HR <65%)

Workout D

Total distance: 1,900 yd

Warm-up: EZ 600 yd (HR <65%)

FA 6 × 100 yd, leaving every 2:30 (HR 80–90%)

Rest 1:00

FA 5 × 50 yd, leaving every 1:10 (HR 80–90%)

Rest 1:00

FA 6 × 25 yd, leaving every 0:35 (HR 80–90%)

Cool-down: EZ 300 yd choice (HR <65%)

Workout E

Total distance: 3,250 yd

Warm-up: EZ 600 yd (HR <65%)

Ladder up and ladder down alternate pull, no rest, EZ (25, 50, 75, 100, 125, 150, 175, 200, 225, 225, 200, 175, 150, 125, 100, 75, 50, 25) (HR <75%)

FA 4 × 25 yd, leaving every 0:35 (HR 80 to 90%)

Cool-down: EZ 300 yd choice (HR <65%)

Workout F

Total distance: 2,950 yd

Warm-up: EZ 600 yd (HR <65%)

MO 6 × 100 yd free with 25 yd kick (total 125 yd) (HR <75%)

EZ 5 × 100 yd EZ alternated with MO 5 × 100 yd fast (HR <75% for EZ, 80–90% for MO)

Rest 2:00

EZ 6 × 25 yd easy alternated with MO 6 × 25 yd fast (HR <75% for EZ, 80–90% for MO)

Cool-down: EZ 300 yd choice (HR <65%)

Workout G

Total distance: 2,800 yd

Warm-up: EZ 600 yd (HR <65%)

FA 5 × 200 yd, complete in 5:00 (HR 80–90%)

Rest 2:00

FA 5 × 100 yd, leaving every 2:30 (HR 80–90%)

Rest 2:00

FA 5 × 50 yd, leaving every 1:10 (HR 80–90%)

Rest 1:00

FA 6 × 25 yards, leaving every 0:35 (HR 80–90%)

Cool-down: EZ 300 yd choice (HR <65%)

Workout H

Total distance: 3,300 yd

Warm-up: EZ 600 yd (HR <65%)

MO pull 600 yd (HR <80%)

EZ swim 600 yd (HR <75%)

MO pull 600 yd (HR <80%)

EZ swim 600 yd (HR <75%)

Cool-down: EZ 300 yd choice (HR <65%)

Workout I

Total distance: 4,250 yd

Warm-up: EZ 600 yd (HR <65%)

Ladder up and ladder down alternate pull, no rest, MO (25, 50, 75, 100, 125, 150, 175, 200, 225, 225, 200, 175, 150, 125, 100, 75, 50, 25) (HR <80%)

EZ 5 × 100 yd EZ alternated with MO 5 × 100 yd fast (HR <75% for EZ, 80–90% for MO)

FA 4 × 25 yd, leaving every 0:35 (HR 80–90%)

Cool-down: EZ 300 yd choice (HR <65%)

Level 3

Congratulations! You are now ready to progress to level 3 (table 12.4). The goal of the level 3 program is to promote economy and speed by working in heart rate training zones 3 (FA) and 4 (VF).

TABLE 12.4 Level 3 Swimming Training Program				
Week	Mon.	Tues.	Wed.	Thurs.	Fri.
1	A (2,950 yd)	B (3,250 yd)	C (1,950 yd)	D (2,525 yd)	E (2,900 yd)
2	A (2,950 yd)	B (3,250 yd)	C (1,950 yd)	D (2,525 yd)	E (2,900 yd)
3	F (3,400 yd)	B (3,250 yd)	C (1,950 yd)	D (2,525 yd)	A (2,950 yd)
4	TT (2,550 yd)	C (1,950 yd)	Rest	B (3,250 yd)	C (1,950 yd)
5	B (3,250 yd)	F (3,400 yd)	Rest	C (1,950 yd)	F (3,400 yd)
6	B (3,250 yd)	Rest	C (1,950 yd)	Rest	TT (2,550 yd)

See chapter text for descriptions of workouts A through F. For English-to-metric conversions, visit www.worldwidemetric.com/measurements.html.

KEY:

TT: Time trial

For the time trial (TT in table 12.4), warm up for 600 yards (548.6 m) at an easy pace (HR <65%) and then swim 1,650 yards (1,509 m) and time your effort. After 1,650 yards, cool down by swimming 300 yards (274.3 m) at an easy pace (HR <65%). Record your result.

Workout A

Total distance: 2,950 yd

Warm-up: EZ 600 yd (HR <65%)

FA 5 × 200 yd alternate pull, complete in 5:00 (HR 80–90%); use a pull buoy for the second and fourth sets

Rest 2:00

FA 6 × 100 yd alternate pull, leaving every 2:30 (HR 80–90%); use a pull buoy for the second, fourth, and sixth sets

Rest 2:00

VF 6 × 50 yd, leaving every 1:00 (HR 90–100%)

Rest 1:00

VF 6 × 25 yd, leaving every 0:30 (HR 90–100%)

Rest 1:00

Cool-down: EZ 300 yd choice (HR <65%)

Workout B

Total distance: 3,250 yd

Warm-up: EZ 600 yd (HR <65%)

Ladder up and ladder down alternate pull, no rest, EZ (25, 50, 75, 100, 125, 150, 175, 200, 225, 225, 200, 175, 150, 125, 100, 75, 50, 25) (HR <75%)

VF 4 × 25 yd, leaving every 0:30 (HR 90–100%)

Rest 1:00

Cool-down: EZ 300 yd choice (HR <65%)

Workout C

Total distance: 1,950 yd

Warm-up: EZ 600 yd (HR <65%)

VF 6 × 100 yd, leaving every 2:20 (HR 90–100%)

Rest 1:00

VF 6 × 50 yd, leaving every 1:05 (HR 90–100%)

Rest 1:00

VF 6 × 25, leaving every 0:30 (HR 90–100%)

Rest 1:00

Cool down: EZ 300 yd choice (HR <65%)

Workout D

Total distance: 2,525 yd

Warm-up: EZ 600 yd (HR <65%)

FA 5 × 100 yd free with 25 yd kick (total 125 yd) (HR 80–90%)

Rest 2:00

EZ 5 × 50 yd easy alternated with MO 5 × 50 yd fast (HR <75% for EZ, 80–90% for MO)

EZ 6 × 25 yd easy alternated with VF 6 × 25 yd fast (HR <75% for EZ, 90–100% for MO)

Rest 2:00

EZ 4 × 25 yd, leaving every 0:30 (HR <65%)

Rest 1:00

EZ 4 × 25yd, leaving every 0:30 (HR <65%)

Cool-down: EZ 300 yd choice (HR <65%)

Workout E

Total distance: 2,900 yd

Warm-up: EZ 600 yd (HR <65%)

FA 10 × 100 yd, leaving every 2:15 (HR 80–90%)

Rest 1:00

FA 10 × 50 yd, leaving every 1:05 (HR 80–90%)

FA 4 × 125 (swim 100 yd, kick 25 yd per set) (HR 80–90%)

Rest 1:00

Cool-down: EZ 300 yd (HR <65%)

Workout F

Total distance: 3,400 yd

Warm-up: EZ 600 yd (HR <65%)

EZ pull 500 yd (HR <75%)

EZ swim 500 yd (HR <75%)

EZ pull 500 yd (HR <75%)

EZ swim 500 yd (HR <75%)

EZ pull 500 yd (HR <75%)

Cool-down: EZ 300 yd choice (HR <65%)

Bonus Triathlon Training

Many triathletes want to swim train specifically for the triathlon. Perhaps they believe that they are weakest in the swim, or perhaps they just don't want their final time resting on how well they perform in the water. Whatever the reason, swim training is a key part of triathlon training. Don't overlook it.

Table 12.5 presents a four-week program for an 800-yard (731.5 m) swim as part of a sprint triathlon and is designed for a beginner. Table 12.6 presents a six-week program for a slightly longer triathlon swim of 1,500 yards

TABLE 12.5 Four-Week 800-Yard Triathlon Swimming Training Program

Week	Mon.	Wed.	Fri.
1	500 yd EZ	500 yd EZ	550 yd EZ
2	550 yd EZ	600 yd EZ	650 yd EZ
3	650 yd EZ	700 yd EZ	750 yd EZ
4	750 yd EZ	800 yd EZ	800 yd EZ

This program is built on three swimming days per week to allow for other training activities.
For English-to-metric conversions, visit www.worldwidemetric.com/measurements.html.

KEY:

EZ: heart rate zone 1

TABLE 12.6 Six-Week 1,500-Yard Triathlon Swimming Training Program

Week	Mon.	Wed.	Fri.
1	800 yd EZ	850 yd EZ	900 yd EZ
2	900 yd EZ	950 yd EZ	1,000 yd EZ
3	1,000 yd EZ	1,050 yd EZ	1,100 yd EZ
4	1,100 yd EZ	1,150 yd EZ	1,200 yd EZ
5	1,250 yd EZ	1,300 yd EZ	1,350 yd EZ
6	1,400 yd EZ	1,450 yd EZ	1,500 yd EZ

This program is built on three swimming days per week and assumes you can already complete an 800-yard swim.
For English-to-metric conversions, visit www.worldwidemetric.com/measurements.html.

KEY:

EZ: heart rate zone 1

(1,371.6 m). Although both distances are less than the 1,650 yards (1,509 m) you will be prepared to swim after the level 1 program, these bonus programs are important because they help you prepare for the swimming aspect of the triathlon while allowing time for training in running and cycling as well. For more on total triathlon training, see chapter 13.

Continuing Your Training

Congratulations. You have laid the foundations of a solid swimming program that will allow you to easily progress to longer distances such as the 2.4-mile (3.9 km) swim of an Ironman triathlon. This progression is straightforward and simply requires an increase in distance. Remember this rule of thumb: Distance should not increase by more than 10 percent over a two- to three-week period. Alternatively, if you are happy with your current level of fitness, you can simply repeat the workouts. If you want to go faster as opposed to farther, reduce the interval times or rest periods between sets. This will make the workouts harder but also improve your overall fitness and speed.

CHAPTER 13

Triathlon

Training for triathlons is one of our favorite programming challenges. Between us, we have done our fair share of events from 5Ks to Ironman, and so we have a few uncanny insights for you. We believe that training for a triathlon can be more enjoyable and less stressful than training for any single endurance event. If you're training for a marathon, all you do is run, but with the triathlon, you get to mix it up and benefit immensely from cross-training. You also have more variability from the environmental stimulus, which can be of great benefit mentally. The cross-training for triathlons also reduces the risk of injury because your body can get more rest than from a single activity training program. However, do not be lured into a false sense of security about triathlons. They present unique challenges from a fitness, neuromuscular, and nutritional point of view. They also force you to recognize your strengths and weaknesses across all three sports, and in some cases, you will find you may need a program that is focused on one of the activities a little more than the others.

One interesting observation about triathlons is that people come from a mix of backgrounds. Some are strong cyclists, some are strong runners, and some are strong swimmers. The lucky few are strong in all three disciplines. Then there are those with no background in any sport who decide to try all three at once.

We need to set a few things straight before going much further. Like single endurance sports, triathlons come in varying distances. In general, there are four recognized triathlon race distances, each approximately double that of the event that comes before it. Table 13.1 is a summary of triathlon distances.

Your first challenge is to select the distance you want to do. Common sense may tell you to begin with the sprint because it is the shortest. However, even a moderately conditioned athlete will take 80 to 90 minutes to complete the sprint. If you are already a seasoned endurance athlete, you may choose to

TABLE 13.1 Triathlon Event Distances

Event	Swim (miles)	Bike (miles)	Run (miles)	Total (miles)
Sprint	0.5	14	3.1	17.6
Olympic	0.9	28	6.2	35.1
Half Ironman	1.2	56	13.1	70.3
Full Ironman	2.4	112	26.2	140.2

dive right in at the Olympic or half Ironman distance. Regardless of your current fitness level, first look to our guidelines for help in deciding where to start. Where you start also will determine your progressions and help ensure a safe and injury-free training program.

Before starting your program, you need to assess your fitness as you would do for any single discipline. For that we recommend assessing yourself in running, cycling, and swimming, using the criteria presented in chapters 10, 11, and 12. From there you'll have a sense of where to start in terms of your triathlon training. Essentially, you'll be able to start at the best level you test at for any discipline.

Determining Your Running, Swimming, and Cycling Training Zones

In chapter 2 and the previous chapters on running, cycling, and swimming, we described the process of determining the heart rate zones for these three sports. Remember, you'll want to try as much as possible to calculate a maximum heart rate for each activity and therefore will have three training zones, one for each sport. These numbers might actually be the same or similar, though this is unlikely. In any case, at least you will have gone through the steps to determine accurate numbers.

Choosing a Training Program

If you are a novice with limited endurance experience in running, cycling, or swimming but you are healthy with no injury concerns, go ahead and line up for the sprint triathlon distance. You should be able to bang this out pretty quickly and then do a couple more for experience before declaring your Olympic distance aspirations. Training to complete a sprint should take 8 to 12 weeks even if you start from scratch.

If you are not a novice but are a fit enthusiast who runs three or four times a week for 4 to 5 miles (6.4 to 8 km) at a time, you are already halfway to completing the Olympic distance triathlon. If this describes you, we would put you into a category we describe as biking or swimming focused—because

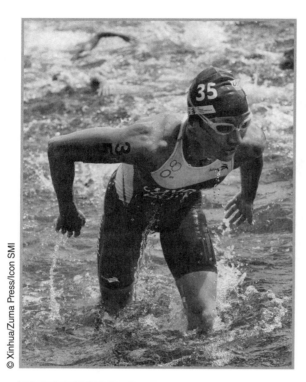

Xinhua/Zuma Press/Icon SMI

Training for a triathlon presents unique challenges. Start by assessing your fitness in all three disciplines.

you have a running background but need some work on the bike and the swim. The big challenge here is tying them all together (especially challenging is the bike-to-run transition).

Once you have a few Olympic triathlons under your belt, you have paved the way for the half Ironman. Be careful, though; there is a significant jump in demands from the Olympic distance to the half Ironman. The half Ironman is not necessarily more complex, but it does require more time for training and conditioning. The same also holds true for the big kahuna, the full Ironman. Table 13.2 shows the typical number of training hours, averaged across the entire training program, someone might put in for each event distance. This table can guide you in selecting an event according to time commitment because we all have real jobs for the rest of the week. For the most part, this is what dictates how much training time we have.

Note that the maximum hours per week noted in table 13.2 are normally achieved at the height of your training programs, whereas the minimum number of hours usually occur just when the program begins or during a recovery week.

One more question is important to consider before choosing a training program, especially in relation to the sprint and Olympic distances: Are you significantly overweight? That is, do you need to drop body weight to do your event? If so, this will really determine the intensity and duration of the

TABLE 13.2 Training Hours per Event Distance				
	Sprint	**Olympic**	**Half Ironman**	**Full Ironman**
Days per week	4 to 6	4 to 6	5 to 7	6 or 7
Minimum hours per week	3 or 4	4 or 5	5 to 7	7 to 9
Maximum hours per week	6 or 7	7 or 8	10 to 12	16 to 19

first four to six weeks of your program. The simple program for the shorter races is based on 12 weeks. However, if you need to drop weight, you will need to add at least four weeks of slow distance work for approximately four to six hours per week before starting the 12-week program.

The programs presented in this chapter are focused on getting you to the finish line with an element of comfort. The programs progress from the sprint to the Olympic distance event. These programs are real programs developed for athletes based on fitness testing in a university laboratory. In other words, we are working from an athlete's true maximum heart rate and training zones.

One last piece of important information that we need to discuss relates to variations in exercise heart rates among different activities. For example, maximum heart rate is different for the same person running, cycling, or swimming. Therefore, you must make accommodations when deciding your heart rate training zone for a particular workout for a particular activity. For example, you might do a steady-state workout in the pool at 30 bpm less than you do a steady-state running workout. Triathletes are advised to have heart rate data for each activity, and then to calculate their training zones and thresholds for all three activities. This increases the accuracy of the overall training program. Look at table 13.3 for an illustration of target training zones and variation in numbers among activities.

TABLE 13.3 Running and Biking Heart Rate (HR) Zones

Zone	Running HR	Biking HR
1	117–138	111–129
2	139–156	130–148
3	157–174	149–165
4	175 or more	166 or more

Level 1: Beginner Sprint Triathlon Training Program

The level 1 program (table 13.4) is for a moderately fit 18- to 35-year-old with no health issues and no real competency in any sport. It also assumes no significant health risk factors. Try to do the exercises in order even if you take a break between them. All running and biking sessions are given in minutes; swimming sessions are given in meters. On rest option days, you may do nothing at all or go for a slow swim.

Note: The biking intervals shown in table 13.5 are used in the level 2 and level 3 programs as well.

Week	Mon.	Tues.	Wed.	Thurs.	Fri.	Sat.	Sun.
		TABLE 13.4 Level 1 Triathlon Training Program: Sprint					
1	Rest option	Bike 45:00 BZ1 Swim 1,200 m	Run 30:00 RZ1	Bike 45:00 BZ1 Swim 1,200 m	Rest option	Bike 30:00 BZ1 Run 30:00 RZ1	Bike >60:00 BZ1–BZ3
2	Rest option	Bike 45:00 BZ1 Swim 1,200 m	Run 30:00 RZ1	Bike 45:00 BZ1 Swim 1,200 m	Rest option	Bike 30:00 BZ1 Run 30:00 RZ1	Bike >60:00 BZ1–BZ3 Run 15:00 RZ1
3	Rest option	Bike 45:00 BZ1 Swim 1,200 m	Run 30:00 RZ1	Bike 45:00 BZ1 Swim 1,200 m	Rest option	Bike 30:00 BZ1 Run 30:00 RZ1	Bike >60:00 BZ1–BZ3 Run 15:00 RZ1
4	Rest option	Bike 45:00 BZ1 Run 15:00 RZ1	Bike 40:00 BZ1	Run 50:00 RZ1 Swim 1,500 m	Rest option	Run 40:00 RZ1 Swim 1,800 m	Bike >60:00 BZ1–BZ3 Run 15:00 RZ1
5	Rest option	Bike 45:00 BZ1 Run 15:00 RZ1	Bike 40:00 BZ1	Run 50:00 RZ1 Swim 1,500 m	Rest option	Run 40:00 RZ1 Swim 1,800 m	Bike >60:00 BZ1–BZ3 Run 15:00 RZ1
6	Rest option	Bike 45:00 BZ1 Run 15:00 RZ1	Bike 40:00 BZ1	Run 50:00 RZ1 Swim 1,500 m	Rest option	Run 40:00 RZ1 Swim 1,000 m	Bike >60:00 BZ1–BZ3 Run 15:00 RZ1
7	Rest option	Bike 30:00 BZ2 Run 30:00 RZ1	Bike 40:00 (20:00 BZ1 and 20:00 BZ2)	Run 30:00 RZ2 Swim 1,000 m	Rest option	Run 30:00 RZ2 Swim 1,200 m	Bike >60:00 BZ1–BZ3 Run 15:00 RZ1
8	Rest option	Bike 30:00 BZ2 Run 30:00 RZ1	Bike 40:00 (20:00 BZ1 and 20:00 BZ2)	Run 30:00 RZ2 Swim 1,000 m	Rest option	Bike 20:00 BZ1 Run 40:00 RZ1	Bike 60:00 1A Run 15:00 RZ1
9	Rest option	Swim 1,500 m Bike 30:00 BZ1	Bike 40:00 (20:00 BZ1 and 20:00 BZ2)	Run 40:00 RZ2 Swim 1,000 m	Rest option	Bike 20:00 BZ1 Run 40:00 RZ1	Bike 60:00 1A Run 20:00 RZ1
10	Rest option	Swim 1,500 m Bike 30:00 BZ1	Bike 40:00 (20:00 BZ1 and 20:00 BZ2)	Run 40:00 RZ2 Swim 1,200 m	Rest option	Run 45:00 (25:00 RZ1 and 20:00 RZ2)	Bike 75:00 1B Run 20:00 RZ1
11	Rest option	Swim 1,500 m Bike 30:00 BZ1	Bike 40:00 (20:00 BZ1 and 20:00 BZ2)	Run 40:00 RZ2 Swim 1,200 m	Rest option	Run 45:00 (25:00 RZ1 and 20:00 RZ2)	Bike 75:00 1B Run 20:00 RZ1
12	Rest option	Swim 1,200 m Bike 30:00 BZ1	Rest option	Run 20:00 RZ2	Bike 30:00 BZ1	Rest	Race

KEY:

BZ: Biking heart rate zone; see table 13.3.
RZ: Running heart rate zone; see table 13.3.
1A, 1B: Biking intervals; see table 13.5.

TABLE 13.5 Triathlon Biking Intervals

Bike 1A		Bike 1B	
Time (min)	Approximate HR (bpm)	Time (min)	Approximate HR (bpm)
0–6	110	0–6	110
6–12	128	6–12	128
12–18	150	12–18	150
18–24	128	18–24	128
24–30	150	24–30	150
30–36	128	30–36	128
36–40	160 or more	36–42	160 or more
40–46	128	42–48	128
46–50	160 or more	48–54	150
50–60	110	54–60	128
		60–66	160 or more
		66–75	110

For the sprint training program (level 1): All intervals at 75–85 rpm.
For the Olympic training programs (level 2): All intervals at 80–90 rpm.
For the half Ironman training program (level 3): All intervals at 80–90 rpm.

Level 2: Olympic Distance Triathlon Training Programs

The first level 2 program (table 13.6) is a progression from the sprint triathlon program, assuming success in the sprint triathlon. Note the added volume and intensity changes from the sprint program. Do all sessions in order even if you take a break between them. All running and biking sessions are given in minutes; swimming sessions are given in meters. On rest option days, you may do nothing at all or go for a slow swim. End all bike rides by incrementally raising your intensity. Increase work rate by 30 to 50 watts every 30 seconds until failure. For the biking intervals, refer back to table 13.5.

The second level 2 program (table 13.7) is a running-focused Olympic distance triathlon training program. It is for those who are competent in both swimming and cycling, but weak in running. The changes from the original Olympic program are bolded. Basically, our philosophy for running-focused programs is to do at least one extra session per week and tag an additional 30 minutes (in 10-minute increments) on to running sessions. If you are biking or swimming challenged, make these adjustments to the initial program using the same logic.

Do all sessions in order even if you take a break between them. All running and biking sessions are given in minutes; swimming sessions are given in meters. On rest option days, you may do nothing at all or go for a slow swim. End all bike rides by incrementally raising your intensity. Increase work rate by 30 to 50 watts every 30 seconds until failure. For the biking intervals, refer back to table 13.5.

TABLE 13.6 Level 2 Triathlon Training Program: Olympic Distance

Week	Mon.	Tues.	Wed.	Thurs.	Fri.	Sat.	Sun.
1	Rest option	Bike 60:00 BZ1 (max last 5:00) Swim 1,200 m	Run 45:00 RZ1	Bike 60:00 BZ1 Swim 1,200 m	Run 30:00 RZ2 Swim 2,500 m	Bike 30:00 BZ1 Run 30:00 RZ1	Bike >90:00 BZ1–BZ3
2	Rest option	Bike 60:00 BZ1 (max last 5:00) Swim 1,200 m steady swim	Run 45:00 RZ1	Bike 60:00 BZ1 Swim 1,200 m steady swim	Run 30:00 RZ2 Swim 2,500 m	Bike 30:00 BZ1 Run 30:00 RZ1	Bike >90:00 BZ1–BZ3 Run 15:00 RZ1
3	Rest option	Bike 60:00 BZ1 (max last 5:00) Swim 1,200 m	Run 45:00 RZ1	Bike 60:00 BZ1 Swim 1,200 m	Run 30:00 RZ2 Swim 2,500 m	Bike 30:00 BZ1 Run 30:00 RZ1	Bike >90:00 BZ1–BZ3 Run 15:00 RZ1
4	Rest option	Bike 45:00 BZ1 Run 15:00 RZ1	Bike 60:00 BZ1	Run 50:00 RZ1 Swim 1,500 m	Bike 60:00 1A Swim 1,000 m	Run 60:00 RZ1 Swim 1,800 m	Bike >90:00 BZ1–BZ3 Run 15:00 RZ1
5	Rest option	Bike 45:00 BZ1 Run 15:00 RZ1	Bike 60:00 BZ1	Run 50:00 RZ1 Swim 1,500 m	Bike 60:00 1A Swim 1,000 m	Run 60:00 RZ1 Swim 1,800 m	Bike >90:00 BZ1–BZ3 Run 15:00 RZ1
6	Rest option	Bike 45:00 BZ1 Run 15:00 RZ1	Bike 60:00 BZ1	Run 50:00 RZ1 Swim 1,500 m	Bike 60:00 1A Swim 1,000 m	Run 60:00 RZ1 Swim 1,000 m	Bike >90:00 BZ1–BZ3 Run 15:00 RZ1
7	Rest option	Bike 30:00 BZ2 Run 30:00 RZ1	Bike 60:00 (30:00 BZ1 and 30:00 BZ2)	Run 30:00 RZ2 Swim 1,000 m steady swim	Bike 75:00 1B Swim 1,000 m steady swim	Run 30:00 RZ2 Swim 2,000 m	Bike >90:00 BZ1–BZ3 Run 15:00 RZ1
8	Rest option	Bike 30:00 BZ2 Run 30:00 RZ1	Bike 60:00 (30:00 BZ1 and 30:00 BZ2)	Run 30:00 RZ2 Swim 1,000 m	Bike 75:00 1B Swim 1,000 m	Bike 20:00 BZ1 Run 60:00 RZ1	Bike >90:00 BZ1–BZ3 Run 15:00 RZ1
9	Rest option	Swim 2,500 m Bike 30:00 BZ1	Bike 60:00 (30:00 BZ1 and 30:00 BZ2)	Run 40:00 RZ2 Swim 1,000 m	Bike 75:00 1B Swim 1,000 m	Bike 20:00 BZ1 Run 60:00 RZ1	Bike >90 BZ1–BZ3 Run 20:00 RZ1
10	Rest option	Swim 2,500 m Bike 30:00 BZ1	Bike 60:00 (20:00 BZ1 and 40:00 BZ2)	Run 40:00 RZ2 Swim 1,200 m	Bike 75:00 1B Run 20:00 RZ1	Run 75:00 (20:00 RZ1, 30:00 RZ2, 25:00 RZ1)	Bike >90:00 BZ1–BZ3 Run 20:00 RZ1 Swim 2,000 m
11	Rest option	Swim 2,500 m Bike 30:00 BZ1	Bike 60:00 (20:00 BZ1 and 40:00 BZ2)	Run 40:00 RZ2 Swim 1,200 m	Bike 75:00 1B Run 20:00 RZ1	Run 75:00 (20:00 RZ1, 30:00 RZ2, 25:00 RZ1)	Bike >90:00 BZ1–BZ3 Run 20:00 RZ1 Swim 2,000 m
12	Rest option	Swim 1,200 m	Bike 30:00 BZ1	Run 20:00 RZ2	Rest	Rest	Race

KEY:

BZ: Biking heart rate zone; see table 13.3.
RZ: Running heart rate zone; see table 13.3.
1A, 1B: Biking intervals; see table 13.5.

TABLE 13.7 Level 2 Triathlon Training Program: Olympic Distance With Running Focus

Week	Mon.	Tues.	Wed.	Thurs.	Fri.	Sat.	Sun.
1	Rest option	Bike 60:00 BZ1 (max last 5:00) Swim 1,200 m	Run 60:00 RZ1	Bike 60:00 BZ1 Swim 1,200 m	Run 40:00 RZ2 Swim 2,500 m	Bike 30:00 BZ1 Run 40:00 RZ1	Bike >90:00 BZ1–BZ3
2	Rest option	Bike 60:00 BZ1 (max last 5:00) Swim 1,200 m steady swim	Run 60:00 RZ1	Bike 60:00 BZ1 Swim 1,200 m steady swim	Run 40:00 RZ2 Swim 2,500 m	Bike 30:00 BZ1 Run 40:00 RZ1	Bike >80:00 BZ1–BZ3 Run 25:00 RZ1
3	Rest option	Bike 60:00 BZ1 (max last 5:00) Swim 1,200 m	Run 60:00 RZ1	Bike 60:00 BZ1 Swim 1,200 m	Run 40:00 RZ2 Swim 2,500 m	Bike 30:00 BZ1 Run 40:00 RZ1	Bike >80:00 BZ1–BZ3 Run 25:00 RZ1
4	Rest option	Bike 45:00 BZ1 Run 15:00 RZ1	Run 60:00 RZ1	Run 50:00 RZ1 Swim 1,500 m	Bike 60:00 1A Swim 1,000 m	Run 75:00 RZ1 Swim 1,800 m	Bike >80:00 BZ1–BZ3 Run 25:00 RZ1
5	Rest option	Bike 45:00 BZ1 Run 15:00 RZ1	Bike 60:00 BZ1	Run 50:00 RZ1 Swim 1,500 m	Bike 60:00 1A Swim 1,000 m	Run 75:00 RZ1 Swim 1,800 m	Bike >80:00 BZ1–BZ3 Run 25:00 RZ1
6	Rest option	Bike 45:00 BZ1 Run 15:00 RZ1	Bike 60:00 BZ1	Run 50:00 RZ1 Swim 1,500 m	Bike 60:00 1A Swim 1,000 m	Run 75:00 RZ1 Swim 1,000 m	Bike >80:00 BZ1–BZ3 Run 25:00 RZ1
7	Rest option	Bike 30:00 BZ2 Run 30:00 RZ1	Bike 60:00 (30:00 BZ1 and 30:00 BZ2)	Run 40:00 RZ2 Swim 1,000 m steady swim	Bike 75:00 1B Swim 1,000 m steady swim	Run 30:00 RZ2 Swim 2,000 m	Bike >80:00 BZ1–BZ3 Run 25:00 RZ1
8	Rest option	Bike 30:00 BZ2 Run 30:00 RZ1	Bike 60:00 (30:00 BZ1 and 30:00 BZ2)	Run 40:00 RZ2 Swim 1,000 m	Bike 75:00 1B Swim 1,000 m	Bike 20:00 BZ1 Run 60:00 RZ1	Bike >80:00 BZ1–BZ3 Run 25:00 RZ1
9	Rest option	Swim 2,500 m Bike 30:00 BZ1	Bike 60:00 (30:00 BZ1 and 30:00 BZ2)	Run 50:00 RZ2 Swim 1,000 m	Bike 75:00 1B Swim 1,000 m	Bike 20:00 BZ1 Run 60:00 RZ1	Bike >90:00 BZ1–BZ3 Run 20:00 RZ1
10	Rest option	Swim 2,500 m Bike 30:00 BZ1	Bike 60:00 (20:00 BZ1 and 40:00 BZ2)	Run 50:00 RZ2 Swim 1,200 m	Bike 75:00 1B Run 20:00 RZ1	Run 75:00 (20:00 RZ1, 30:00 RZ2, 25:00 RZ1)	Bike >90:00 BZ1–BZ3 Run 20:00 RZ1 Swim 2,000 m

(continued)

TABLE 13.7 *(continued)*

Week	Mon.	Tues.	Wed.	Thurs.	Fri.	Sat.	Sun.
11	Rest option	Swim 2,500 m Bike 30:00 BZ1	Bike 60:00 (20:00 BZ1 and 40:00 BZ2)	Run 50:00 RZ2 Swim 1,200 m	Bike 75:00 1B Run 20:00 RZ1	Run 75:00 (20:00 RZ1, 30:00 RZ2, 25:00 RZ1)	Bike >90:00 BZ1–BZ3 Run 20:00 RZ1 Swim 2,000 m
12	Rest option	Swim 1,200 m	Bike 30:00 BZ1	Run 20:00 RZ2	Rest	Rest	Race

KEY:

BZ: Biking heart rate zone; see table 13.3.
RZ: Running heart rate zone; see table 13.3.
1A, 1B: Biking intervals; see table 13.5.

Level 3: Half Ironman Training Program

Advancing to the next level of training (half Ironman) is more complex. For that reason, we advise you to work closely with a knowledgeable coach who can create a program specifically for you, even more important if you seek to attempt the full Ironman.

The half Ironman and full Ironman distances are considerable undertakings requiring a minimum of five months of basic training for the half Ironman and 9 to 12 months for the full Ironman. In this chapter we provide a sample template for a half Ironman only (table 13.8) and again advise you to seek personal, knowledgeable help for the big kahuna.

The half Ironman has some prerequisites. As a general rule you should not even think about attempting a half Ironman unless you can comfortably perform an Olympic distance event and swim for 45 minutes, run for 60 minutes, and bike for 90 minutes consistently and comfortably. It would be advantageous if you could put these three together back-to-back regardless of the speed at which you do them. Notice that we recommend dedicating a minimum of 20 weeks to a half Ironman training program.

In this program, only swimming distance is provided. Most swimming programs address more specific stroke and speed development and use a lot of variations in intervals. This would be individualized for you if you worked with a personal trainer. You also can look at chapter 12 for more detailed swimming workouts.

Entering into the half Ironman distance has another set of issues such as nutrition. We advise that you get personal help with this aspect of training.

TABLE 13.8 Level 3 Triathlon Training Program: Half Ironman Distance

Week	Mon.	Tues.	Wed.	Thurs.	Fri.	Sat.	Sun.
1	Rest option	Bike 75:00 BZ1 (max last 5:00) Swim 1,800 m	Run 60:00 RZ1	Bike 75:00 BZ1 (max last 5:00) Swim 1,800 m	Run 40:00 RZ2 Swim 2,500 m	Bike 40:00 BZ1 Run 50:00 RZ1	Bike >90:00 BZ1–BZ3
2	Rest option	Bike 75:00 BZ1 (max last 5:00) Swim 1,800 m	Run 60:00 RZ1	Bike 75:00 BZ1 (max last 5:00) Swim 1,800 m	Run 40:00 RZ2 Swim 2,500 m steady swim	Bike 40:00 BZ1 Run 50:00 RZ1	Bike >90:00 BZ1–BZ3 Run 25:00 RZ1
3	Rest option	Bike 75:00 BZ1 (max last 5:00) Swim 1,800 m	Run 60:00 RZ1	Bike 75:00 BZ1 (max last 5:00) Swim 1,800 m	Run 40:00 RZ2 Swim 2,500 m	Bike 40:00 BZ1 Run 50:00 RZ1	Bike >90:00 BZ1–BZ3 R25 RZ1
4	Rest option	Bike 60:00 BZ1 Run 15:00 RZ1	Run 60:00 RZ1	Run 50:00 RZ1 Swim 2,500 m	Bike 60:00 1A Swim 1,500 m	Run 75:00 RZ1 Swim 2,000 m	Bike >90:00 BZ1–BZ3 Run 25:00 RZ1
5	Rest option	Bike 60:00 BZ1 Run 15:00 RZ1	Bike 60:00 BZ1	Run 50:00 RZ1 Swim 2,500 m	Bike 60:00 1A Swim 1,500 m	Run 75:00 RZ1 Swim 2,000 m	Bike >120:00 BZ1–BZ3 Run 25:00 RZ1
6	Rest option	Bike 60:00 BZ1 Run 15:00 RZ1	Bike 60:00 BZ1	Run 50:00 RZ1 Swim 2,500 m	Bike 60:00 1A Swim 1,500 m	Run 75:00 RZ1 Swim 2,000 m	Bike >120:00 BZ1–BZ3 Run 25:00 RZ1
7	Rest option	Bike 60:00 BZ2 Run 40:00 RZ1	Bike 90:00 (60:00 BZ1 and 30:00 BZ2)	Run 60:00 RZ2 Swim 1,500 m steady swim	Bike 75:00 1B Swim 1,500 m steady swim	Run 30:00 RZ2 Swim 2,000 m	Bike >120:00 BZ1–BZ3 Run 25:00 RZ1
8	Rest option	Bike 60:00 BZ2 Run 30:00 RZ1	Bike 90:00 (60:00 BZ1 and 30:00 BZ2)	Run 60:00 RZ2 Swim 1,500 m	Bike 75:00 1B Swim 1,500 m	Bike 30:00 BZ1 Run 60:00 RZ1	Bike >120:00 BZ1–BZ3 Run 25:00 RZ1
9	Rest option	Swim 2,500 m Bike 30:00 BZ1	Bike 90:00 (60:00 BZ1 and 30:00 BZ2)	Run 60:00 RZ2 Swim 1,500 m	Bike 75:00 1B Swim 1,500 m	Bike 30:00 BZ1 Run 60:00 RZ1	Bike >120:00 BZ1–BZ3 Run 30:00 RZ1
10	Rest option	Swim 2,500 m Bike 30:00 BZ1	Bike 90:00 (60:00 BZ1 and 30:00 BZ2)	Run 120:00	Bike 75:00 1B Swim 1,500 m	Rest	Bike >120:00 BZ1–BZ3 Run 20:00 RZ1 Swim 2,000 m

(continued)

TABLE 13.8 *(continued)*

Week	Mon.	Tues.	Wed.	Thurs.	Fri.	Sat.	Sun.
11	Rest option	Swim 2,500 m Bike 30:00 BZ1	Bike 90:00 (60:00 BZ1 and 30:00 BZ2)	Run 120:00	Bike 75:00 1B Swim 1,500 m	Rest	Bike >120:00 BZ1–BZ3 Run 20:00 RZ1 Swim 2,000 m
12	Rest option	Swim 1,200 m	Bike 30:00 BZ1	Run 20:00 RZ2	Rest	Rest	Bike >180:00 BZ1 Run 20:00 RZ1 Swim 2,000 m
13	Rest option	Swim 2,000 m	Bike 60:00 BZ1 Run 30:00 RZ1	Rest	Run 40:00 RZ2	Bike 60:00 BZ1 Swim 2,000 m	Bike >180:00 BZ1–BZ3 Run 20:00 RZ1 Swim 2,000 m
14	Rest option	Rest option	Bike 60:00 BZ1 Swim 2,000 m	Run 60:00 RZ1	Bike 75:00 1B Run 20:00 RZ1	Run 120:00 RZ1	Bike >180:00 BZ1
15	Rest option	Bike 60:00 BZ1 Swim 3,000 m	Bike 60:00 BZ1 Run 20:00 RZ1	Rest	Run 120:00 RZ1	Rest	Bike >240:00 BZ1 Run 10:00 RZ1
16	Rest option	Bike 60:00 BZ1 Swim 3,000 m	Rest	Run 150:00 RZ1	Rest	Rest	Bike >240:00 BZ1 Run 30:00 RZ1
17	Rest option	Rest option	Bike 60:00 BZ1 Swim 3,000 m	Bike 60:00 BZ1 Run 30:00 RZ1	Swim 3,000 m	Rest	Bike >240:00 BZ1 Run 30:00 RZ1
18	Rest option	Rest option	Run 120:00 BZ1	Bike 60:00 BZ1 Run 60:00 RZ1	Swim 3,000 m	Rest	Swim 2,000 m Bike 90:00 BZ1 Run 30:00 RZ1
19	Rest option	Swim 3,000 m	Bike 60:00 BZ1 Run 60:00 RZ1	Swim 2,000 m Bike 60:00 BZ1	Rest	Rest	Bike >240:00 BZ1 Run 20:00 RZ1
20	Rest option	Rest	Swim 1,500 m Run 30:00 RZ1	Bike 45:00 BZ1	Rest	Rest	Race

KEY:

BZ: Biking heart rate zone; see table 13.3.
RZ: Running heart rate zone; see table 13.3.
1A, 1B: Biking intervals; see table 13.5.

Continuing Your Training

You now have a spectrum of triathlon training programs based on heart rate training—from the sprint triathlon through the half Ironman. You may have noticed that the sprint and Olympic programs are similar in terms of heart rate training zones and progressions. However, when you do these workouts, you will find that the intensity or work output (speed or watts) is much higher at the same heart rate when you are doing the Olympic program versus the sprint program. This illustrates the beauty of heart rate training—you have an internal regulator that keeps you working honestly. Good record keeping is extremely important. You will be able to track your changes in fitness by watching for that lowering heart rate (or increasing speed) as long as you document those numbers and keep an eye on the monitor. And remember, as a triathlete, you will have this effect occurring on three different levels across three different activities.

Now is the time to decide how content you are with your current level of fitness. If you are happy with where you are, your hard work is done, and you can maintain your fitness by backing off a little bit in terms of both volume and frequency but maintaining a few high-intensity exercise sessions per week. If you want to achieve a higher level of fitness and be more competitive, you have to think about a more structured training regime that focuses more on your abilities as opposed to just your fitness. You probably will want to seek professional help because you will need to think about more specific training sessions that focus on your strengths and weakness instead of a general overall fitness approach. Nutrition will also become more important, as will technique, equipment, and bike fit, among other issues.

CHAPTER 14

Rowing

Like swimming, rowing is a complex skill sport. It is further unique in that the skill set required to row on an indoor rower is very different from the skill set required to row on the water. Indeed, rowing may be one of the most technically difficult of all the dynamic aerobic activities. For that reason, our focus in this chapter will only be on exercise sessions on indoor rowing ergometers because they are widely available and present much less of a technical component. A talented rower can apply the program to on-the-water training as well.

The indoor ergometer has numerous useful features such as split times for 500 meters and wattage, stroke count, and time trial functions that allow you to set your own distance and have it timed by the computer. Before you go too far, familiarize yourself with the basic computer features, especially the 500-meter split function because we use this feature a lot in our program design.

As with all other aerobic exercise programs, knowing where to start can be a challenge. In the case of rowing, we suggest the simple task of rowing 2,000 meters as fast as you can to evaluate your basic fitness level. From there you can determine your basic fitness classification and then identify an appropriate training program. Because 2,000 meters is a very popular indoor and outdoor distance, we also use this distance as a goal race target for the training programs. We have used the same logic and progression that we used in other chapters and have provided three progressions to allow you to achieve an initial goal and then move on to more advanced goals. So let's get started by performing the initial test to determine current fitness levels.

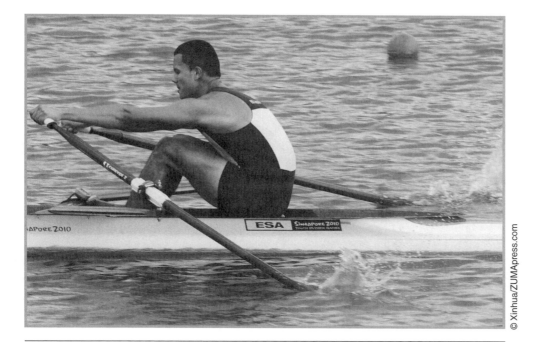

Although rowing is a complex skill, the principles of smart training still apply. Develop a good foundation of endurance and build on it to generate stamina, power, and speed.

Classifying Your Current Fitness Level

To determine your starting point, you need to classify your current level of fitness. Start by performing a 15-minute, moderate warm-up. After the warm-up, perform an all-out 2,000-meter set and record your finishing time.

Based on the results of the rowing test and the data from table 14.1, you can calculate your rowing $\dot{V}O_2max$ using this formula developed by Dr. Hagerman:

$$\dot{V}O_2max = (Y \times 1,000) \setminus body\ weight\ (kg)$$

Use table 14.1 to determine the value of Y based on your finishing time in the 2,000-meter test, your gender, and your weight in kilograms. The table

TABLE 14.1 Determining the Value of Y to Calculate Rowing $\dot{V}O_2max$				
	Females <61.36 kg	**Females >61.36 kg**	**Males <75 kg**	**Males >75 kg**
High training level	Y = 14.6 − (1.5 × time)	Y = 14.9 − (1.5 × time)	Y = 15.1 − (1.5 × time)	Y = 15.7 − (1.5 × time)
Low training level	Y = 10.26 − (0.93 × time)		Y = 10.7 − (0.9 × time)	

depicts two training levels, low and high. The low training level equals fewer than three times per week and applies to noncompetitive rowers (weekly volume <25 k). The high training level equals more than three sessions per week and generally applies to more competitive rowers. Time is in minutes.

For example, if a male rower who weighs 79 kilograms rows 2,000 meters in 8 minutes, the calculation would be as follows:

$$Y = 15.7 - (1.5 \times 8{:}00) = 3.7$$
$$\dot{V}O_2max = (3.7 \times 1,000) / 79\ kg = 46.8\ ml/kg/min$$

Based on this initial fitness test, start your rowing training program at the level indicated. See table 14.2 (if you are male) or table 14.3 (if you are female) to find your fitness category.

TABLE 14.2 Fitness Classifications Based on $\dot{V}O_2max$ Results: Male Athletes

Age	Poor	Fair	Average	Good	Excellent
15–19	≤52	53–57	58–65	66–69	≥70
20–29	≤52	53–59	60–69	70–77	≥78
30–39	≤47	48–53	54–62	63–71	≥72
40–49	≤39	40–43	44–55	56–63	≥64
50–59	≤31	32–37	38–51	52–57	≥58
60–69	≤22	23–30	31–42	43–54	≥55
	Level 1		**Level 2**		**Levels 3 and 4**

Note: Classifications reflect conditioning status for endurance athletes. Data for nonathletes would be much lower.

TABLE 14.3 Fitness Classifications Based on $\dot{V}O_2max$ Results: Female Athletes

Age	Poor	Fair	Average	Good	Excellent
15–19	≤48	49–54	55–61	62–67	≥68
20–29	≤49	50–54	55–62	63–71	≥72
30–39	≤39	40–49	50–55	56–64	≥65
40–49	≤28	29–40	41–48	49–59	≥60
50–59	≤19	20–28	29–40	41–50	≥51
60–69	≤7	8–14	15–25	26–41	≥42
	Level 1		**Level 2**		**Levels 3 and 4**

Note: Classifications reflect conditioning status for endurance athletes. Data for nonathletes would be much lower.

Determining Your Rowing Training Zones

In the process of assessing your current fitness level, you should also collect your heart rate data. Assuming that you give a maximum effort and perform the 2,000-meter test as fast as possible, you should get your true rowing maximum heart rate. Use this number to calculate your various training zones.

The logic for determining maximum heart rate for rowing is essentially the same as the logic for other sports described in other chapters. The main difference is that in rowing the 2,000 m, the exertion is not progressive with multiple stages, so be sure to include a nice, long, and appropriate warm-up.

Chapter 6 provided a test for calculating anaerobic threshold. The problem with the sport of rowing is that if you simply do a 2,000-meter rowing test as fast as you can, you will not be able to determine your anaerobic threshold. To find your anaerobic threshold, you must perform an incremental, or progressive, test to exhaustion and record your heart rate every 30 seconds during the test. For rowing, we suggest a starting pace of 3 minutes per 500 meters, decreasing by 10 seconds per 500 meters for every 2 minutes until you reach a pace of 2 minutes per 500 meters. Once you drop below a 2-minute pace per 500 meters, decrease the pace by 5 seconds instead of 10 seconds per 500 meters every 2 minutes. Most likely you will need someone to record the data for you.

When you look back at the data, draw a chart and determine the stage where HR no longer plateaued after a change in work rate. This is a rough estimate of AT.

Choosing a Training Program

It is important that you start at the right level and spend enough time at the right intensity to develop your basic fitness before you move on to harder work. (Table 14.4 lists the rowing training phases.) Use your 2,000-meter time to help you determine the level and program at which to start. All the programs keep you in a base-building mode for a period of weeks, regardless of your initial level of fitness. You should move up in intensity after establishing a good foundation, regardless of your fitness level. Everyone benefits from a period of base building.

TABLE 14.4 Rowing Training Phases	
Training phase	**Percent MHR**
Phase I: Endurance (EZ)	60–75%
Phase II: Stamina (MO)	75–85%
Phase III: Economy (FA)	85–95%
Phase IV: Speed endurance (VF)	95–100%

Level 1

The zone 1 (Z1) workouts (table 14.5) are very easy and may in fact get boring. Try to stick with them. Use the heart rate monitor and exercise as hard as you like, but you must stay under 75 percent maximum heart rate (MHR). The same logic applies to the zone 2 stamina (MO) workouts. Stay under 85 percent MHR.

Because most people have more time on the weekends, the weekend workouts are longer.

The 2K and 6K workouts are all-out efforts. Finish strong. For the 2K and 6K time trails, warm up by performing a 500-meter split at a 2:40 pace for 5 minutes, then drop to a 2:30 pace for a 500-meter split for an additional 5 minutes, and then a 2:20 pace for a 500-meter split for 5 minutes. Rest for 3 minutes, and then perform the 2K or 6K all out. Record your times for all trials.

The rest days follow harder days of intervals. Use rest days wisely and do nothing strenuous. Unless you are highly trained, we suggest a full rest. If you are highly trained, you might perform a short recovery workout—for example, 30 minutes at less than 65 percent MHR.

The intervals are designed to be hard. They will be uncomfortable. When you perform the intervals A1, A2, and A3, don't worry about your heart rate, but do record it. Use this to document changes in fitness. These intervals will fluctuate between zone 3, economy (FA), and zone 4, speed endurance (VF), and then go back down to zone 1, endurance (EZ), during recovery.

TABLE 14.5 Level 1 Rowing Training Program: Beginner

Week	Mon.	Tues.	Wed.	Thurs.	Fri.	Sat.	Sun.
1	2K TT	EZ 45:00	MO 45:00	Rest	A1	Rest	6K TT
2	Rest	EZ 45:00	MO 45:00	Rest	A1	EZ 60:00	MO 60:00
3	Rest	EZ 45:00	MO 45:00	Rest	A1	EZ 60:00	MO 60:00
4	Rest	EZ 45:00	MO 45:00	Rest	A1	EZ 60:00	MO 60:00
5	Rest	EZ 50:00	A3	Rest	2K TT	EZ 60:00	MO 60:00
6	Rest	EZ 50:00	A3	Rest	A1	Rest	6K TT
7	Rest	EZ 50:00	A3	Rest	A1	EZ 75:00	MO 75:00
8	Rest	EZ 50:00	A3	Rest	A1	EZ 75:00	MO 75:00
9	Rest	EZ 55:00	MO 50:00	Rest	2K TT	EZ 75:00	MO 75:00
10	Rest	EZ 55:00	MO 50:00	Rest	A1	EZ 75:00	MO 75:00
11	Rest	EZ 55:00	MO 50:00	Rest	6K TT	Rest	MO 90:00
12	Rest	EZ 55:00	MO 50:00	Rest	A2	EZ 60:00	2K TT

Goal: Row 2K in less than 9:00. See chapter text for descriptions of interval sessions.

KEY:

TT: Time trial
EZ: Heart rate zone 1
MO: Heart rate zone 2

A1 Interval

Approximately 43:00, excluding warm-up and cool-down

Warm-up: Easy row 10:00 (2:30 to 2:40 500-meter split)

2:20 500-meter split for 6:00

2:30 500-meter split for 6:00

2:15 500-meter split for 6:00

2:30 500-meter split for 6:00

2:10 500-meter split for 6:00

2:30 500-meter split for 5:00

2:05 500-meter split for 3:00

2:30 500-meter split for 3:00

2:00 500-meter split for 2:00 or as long as possible

Recovery cool-down: Easy row 10:00 (2:40 500-meter split)

A2 Interval

Approximately 41:00, excluding warm-up and cool-down

Warm-up: Easy row 10:00 (2:30 to 2:40 500-meter split)

2:25 500-meter split for 15:00

2:15 500-meter split for 7:00

2:25 500-meter split for 7:00

2:10 500-meter split for 2:00

2:20 500-meter split for 2:00

2:25 500-meter split for 2:00

2:05 500-meter split for 2:00

2:25 500-meter split for 2:00

1:55 500-meter split for 2:00 or as long as possible

Recovery cool-down: Easy row 10:00 to 15:00 (less than 2:40 500-meter split)

A3 Interval

Approximately 30:00, excluding warm-up and cool-down

Warm-up: Easy row 15:00 (2:30 to 2:40 500-meter split)

2:25 500-meter split for 5:00

2:20 500-meter split for 5:00

2:15 500-meter split for 5:00

2:10 500-meter split for 5:00

2:05 500-meter split for 5:00

2:00 500-meter split for 5:00

Recovery cool-down: Easy row 10:00 (less than 2:40 500-meter split)

Level 2

Before moving to the level 2 program (table 14.6), you need to ask yourself two questions. First, have you completed level 1? Second, have you met the criteria for level 2 by doing a retest on the 2,000-meter test in less than 9:00? If you redo the 2,000-meter test and fall short, we suggest you repeat the last four weeks of the level 1 program.

For the 2K and 6K time trials, warm up by performing a 2:30 500-meter split for 5 minutes, a 2:20 500-meter split for 5 minutes, and a 2:10 500-meter split for 5 minutes. Then perform the 2K or 6K all out. Record your times for every trial.

TABLE 14.6 Level 2 Rowing Training Program: Intermediate

Week	Mon.	Tues.	Wed.	Thurs.	Fri.	Sat.	Sun.
1	2K TT	EZ 55:00	MO 50:00	Rest	A1	EZ 75:00	MO 75:00
2	Rest	EZ 55:00	MO 50:00	Rest	A1	EZ 75:00	MO 75:00
3	Rest	EZ 55:00	MO 50:00	Rest	A2	Rest	6K TT
4	Rest	EZ 55:00	MO 50:00	Rest	A2	EZ 90:00	MO 90:00
5	Rest	EZ 60:00	A4	Rest	2K TT	EZ 90:00	Rest
6	Rest	EZ 60:00	A4	Rest	A2	EZ 90:00	Rest
7	Rest	EZ 60:00	A4	Rest	A2	EZ 90:00	Rest
8	Rest	EZ 60:00	A4	Rest	A2	Rest	6K TT
9	Rest	MO 45:00	FA 45:00	Rest	2K TT	MO 30:00	A4
10	Rest	MO 45:00	FA 45:00	Rest	A2	MO 30:00	A4
11	Rest	MO 45:00	FA 45:00	Rest	A2	MO 30:00	A4
12	Rest	MO 45:00	Rest	Rest	2K TT	MO 30:00	6K TT

Goal: Row 2K in 0:30 less than previous 2K time. See chapter text for descriptions of intervals.

KEY:

TT: Time trial
EZ: Heart rate zone 1
MO: Heart rate zone 2
FA: Heart rate zone 3

Here are descriptions of the intervals noted in table 14.6:

A1 Interval

Approximately 43:00, excluding warm-up and cool-down

Warm-up: Easy row 15:00 (2:20 to 2:40 500-meter split)

2:10 500-meter split for 6:00

2:25 500-meter split for 6:00

2:05 500-meter split for 6:00

2:25 500-meter split for 6:00

2:00 500-meter split for 6:00

2:25 500-meter split for 5:00

1:55 500-meter split for 3:00

2.25 500-meter split for 3:00

1:50 500-meter split for 2:00

Recovery cool-down: Easy row 10:00 (more than 2:30 500-meter split)

A2 Interval

Approximately 41:00, excluding warm-up and cool-down

Warm-up: Easy row 15:00 (2:20 to 2:40 500-meter split)

2:15 500-meter split for 15:00

2:05 500-meter split for 7:00

2:15 500-meter split for 7:00

2:00 500-meter split for 2:00

2:10 500-meter split for 2:00

2:15 500-meter split for 2:00

1:55 500-meter split for 2:00

2:15 500-meter split for 2:00

1:50 500-meter split for 2:00

Recovery cool-down: Easy row 10:00 to 15:00 (more than 2:30 500-meter split)

A3 Interval

Approximately 30:00, excluding warm-up and cool-down

Warm-up: Easy row 15:00 (2:20 to 2:40 500-meter split)

2:25 500-meter split for 5:00

2:20 500-meter split for 5:00

2:15 500-meter split for 5:00

2:10 500-meter split for 5:00

2:05 500-meter split for 5:00

2:00 500-meter split for 5:00

Recovery cool-down: Easy row 10:00 (more than 2:30 500-meter split)

A4 Interval

Approximately 42:00, excluding warm-up and cool-down

Warm-up: Easy row 15:00 (2:20 to 2:40 500-meter split)

2:25 500-meter split for 6:00

2:20 500-meter split for 6:00

2:15 500-meter split for 6:00

2:10 500-meter split for 6:00

2:05 500-meter split for 6:00

2:00 500-meter split for 6:00

1:55 500-meter split for 6:00

Recovery cool-down: Easy row 10:00 (more than 2:30 500-meter split)

Level 3

Before advancing to level 3 (table 14.7), ask yourself the same two questions you asked when you progressed from level 1 to level 2: Did you complete levels 1 and 2, and did you meet the time requirements for the 2,000-meter test to be classified as advanced? Often, people who come to rowing from other modes of exercise are quite fit. If this situation applies to you, use the criteria time for the 2,000-meter test alone.

For the 2K time trial, warm up by performing a 2:20 500-meter split for 5 minutes, a 2:15 500-meter split for 5 minutes, and a 2:10 500-meter split for 5 minutes. Then perform the 2K all out. Record your times for every trial.

Here are descriptions of the intervals noted in table 14.7:

A1 Interval

Approximately 45:00, excluding warm-up and cool-down

Warm-up: Easy row 15:00 (2:20 to 2:30 500-meter split)

2:00 500-meter split for 8:00

2:15 500-meter split for 6:00

1:55 500-meter split for 6:00

2:15 500-meter split for 6:00

1:50 500-meter split for 6:00

2:15 500-meter split for 5:00

1:45 500-meter split for 5:00

2:15 500-meter split for 3:00

Recovery cool-down: Easy row 3:00 (2:20 500-meter split)

A2 Interval

Approximately 41:00, excluding warm-up and cool-down

Warm-up: Easy row 15:00 (2:20 to 2:30 500-meter split)

2:00 500-meter split for 15:00

1:50 500-meter split for 7:00

2:15 500-meter split for 7:00

2:05 500-meter split for 2:00

TABLE 14.7 Level 3 Rowing Training Program: Advanced

Week	Mon.	Tues.	Wed.	Thurs.	Fri.	Sat.	Sun.
1	2K TT	FA 30:00	EZ 30:00	A1	Rest	EZ 120:00	EZ 60:00
2	Rest	FA 30:00	EZ 60:00	A1	Rest	EZ 120:00	EZ 60:00
3	EZ 60:00	FA 30:00	EZ 60:00	A1	Rest	EZ 120:00	EZ 60:00
4	EZ 60:00	FA 30:00	EZ 30:00	EZ 30:00	Rest	2K TT	Rest
5	EZ 60:00	FA 30:00 VF 5:00	Rest	EZ 60:00	MO 45:00	EZ 120:00	EZ 60:00
6	EZ 60:00	FA 30:00 VF 10:00	Rest	EZ 60:00	MO 45:00	EZ 60:00 MO 60:00	Rest
7	EZ 30:00	FA 30:00 VF 10:00	EZ 30:00	EZ 60:00	MO 60:00	EZ 60:00 MO 60:00	Rest
8	EZ 60:00	FA 30:00 VF 15:00	A2	Rest	MO 60:00	EZ 60:00 MO 60:00	Rest
9	EZ 60:00	A3	A4	EZ 60:00	a.m.: A3 p.m.: EZ 30:00	Rest	A4
10	EZ 60:00	A5	A4	EZ 60:00	a.m.: A5 p.m.: EZ 30:00	Rest	A6
11	EZ 60:00	A6	A2	EZ 60:00	a.m.: 2K TT p.m.: EZ 30:00	Rest	A7
12	EZ 30:00	5K 20:00	Rest	Rest or easy 5K	Rest	Rest	2K TT

Goal: Row 2K in 0:20 less than previous 2K time. See chapter text for descriptions of intervals.

KEY:

TT: Time trial
EZ: Heart rate zone 1
MO: Heart rate zone 2
FA: Heart rate zone 3
VF: Heart rate zone 4

2:00 500-meter split for 2:00

2:15 500-meter split for 2:00

1:55 500-meter split for 2:00

2:15 500-meter split for 2:00

1:50 500-meter split for 2:00

Recovery cool-down: Easy row 10:00 to 15:00 (2:15 to 2:20 500-meter split)

A3 Interval

Approximately 63:00, excluding warm-up and cool-down

Warm-up: Easy row 15:00 (2:20 to 2:30 500-meter split)

2:00 500-meter split for 8:00

2:15 500-meter split for 6:00

1:55 500-meter split for 6:00

2:15 500-meter split for 6:00

1:50 500-meter split for 6:00

2:15 500-meter split for 5:00

1:45 500-meter split for 5:00

2.15 500-meter split for 5:00

1:40 500-meter split for 3:00

2:15 500-meter split for 5:00

1:35 500-meter split for 3:00

2:15 500-meter split for 5:00

Recovery cool-down: Easy row 10:00 to 15:00 (2:15 to 2:20 500-meter split)

A4 Interval

Approximately 42:00, excluding warm-up and cool-down

Warm-up: Easy row 15:00 (2:20 to 2:30 500-meter split)

2:00 500-meter split for 15:00

1:50 500-meter split for 7:00

2:15 500-meter split for 7:00

2:05 500-meter split for 2:00

2:00 500-meter split for 2:00

1:55 500-meter split for 2:00

1:50 500-meter split for 2:00

1:45 500-meter split for 2:00

1:40 500-meter split for 2:00

All-out 1:00

Recovery cool-down: Easy row 5:00 (more than 2:15 500-meter split)

A5 Interval

Approximately 55:00, excluding warm-up and cool-down

Warm-up: Easy row 15:00 (2:20 to 2:30 500-meter split)

1:55 500-meter split for 7:00

2:15 500-meter split for 5:00

1:50 500-meter split for 6:00

2:15 500-meter split for 5:00

1:45 500-meter split for 6:00

2:15 500-meter split for 5:00

1:40 500-meter split for 5:00

2:15 500-meter split for 5:00

1:40 500-meter split for 4:00

2:15 500-meter split for 5:00

1:35 500-meter split for 2:00

Recovery cool-down: Easy row 5:00 (more than 2:15 500-meter split)

A6 Interval

Approximately 42:00, excluding warm-up and cool-down

Warm-up: Easy row 15:00 (2:20 to 2:30 500-meter split)

1:55 500-meter split for 15:00

2:15 500-meter split for 5:00

1:40 500-meter split for 4:00

2:15 500-meter split for 4:00

1:40 500-meter split for 4:00

2:15 500-meter split for 2:00

1:35 500-meter split for 2:00

2:15 500-meter split for 4:00

1:35 500-meter split for 2:00

Recovery cool-down: Easy row 5:00 (more than 2:15 500-meter split)

A7 Interval

Approximately 42:00, excluding warm-up and cool-down

Warm-up: Easy row 15:00 (2:20 to 2:40 500-meter split)

1:35 to 1:38 500-meter split for 3:00

2:15 500-meter split for 4:00 (recovery)

1:35 to 1:38 500-meter split for 3:00

2:15 500-meter split for 4:00 (recovery)

1:35 to 1:38 500-meter split for 3:00

2:15 500-meter split for 4:00 (recovery)

1:35 to 1:38 500-meter split for 3:00

2:15 500-meter split for 4:00 (recovery)

1:35 to 1:38 500-meter split for 3:00

2:15 500-meter split for 4:00 (recovery)

1:35 to 1:38 500-meter split for 3:00

2:15 500-meter split for 4:00 (recovery)

Recovery cool-down: Easy row 5:00 (2:15 500-meter split)

Continuing Your Training

Congratulations on making your way through a lot of training. As with other sports, in rowing, getting fit is the hardest part. Now that you have achieved this, the question is, How happy are you with your fitness level? If you are satisfied, you can simply back off and train about three days per week at the average intensities within your current training level. This will ensure you maintain your fitness. Be sure to retain your intensity as this is the most important component in maintaining fitness. If you want to conquer bigger water, you need to look to more advanced programs that take other elements of performance such as nutrition and technique into account.

CHAPTER 15

Cross-Country Skiing

Thus far, we have covered walking, running, cycling, swimming, the triathlon, and rowing. Cross-country skiing is the last endurance sport we cover. Cross-country skiers have notoriously posted the most impressive numbers in fitness testing of all the endurance athletes. Although there is no doubting the fitness of all top endurance athletes, cross-country, or nordic, skiers reign supreme. Look at table 15.1 for some reported $\dot{V}O_2max$ findings in elite athletes from various sports. Despite the well-recognized names and accomplishments of those in the table, cross-country skiers are a step above everyone else. What is particularly interesting about cross-country skiers from both a physiological and evolutionary point of view is that they have not only improved their performance physiology, but in the last 50-60 years have also surpassed their endurance sport counterparts in improvement percentages.

Running 10K records have dipped below 27 minutes, which represents an improvement of less than 15 percent over the last century. Speed skaters today travel about 25 percent faster than those of a century ago; swimmers fare very well at upward of 40 percent. On the other hand, cross-country skiers have cut race times for the traditional distances of 25K and 50K pretty much in half over the last century. Admittedly, advances in equipment and materials have aided greatly and account for much of the improvement, but changes in training philosophy, high-intensity work, rest, strength training, nutrition, and other factors have also played a major role. These changes occurred in other sports, too, but cross-country skiing has long been on the cutting edge of training methodology, and more to the point, these athletes rely very heavily on heart rate training methodology.

Athlete	Gender	Sport	$\dot{V}O_2$max (ml/kg/min)
Bjorn Daehlie	Male	Cross-country skiing	94.0
Greg LeMond	Male	Cycling	92.5
Miguel Indurain	Male	Cycling	88.0
Lance Armstrong	Male	Cycling	84.0
Steve Prefontaine	Male	Running	84.4
I. Kristiannssen	Female	Running	71.2
Rosa Mota	Female	Running	67.2

TABLE 15.1 $\dot{V}O_2$max Data of Top Endurance Athletes

It would be fair to say that the Scandinavians have pioneered not only heart rate measurement, but also heart rate training and monitoring with cross-country skiers. The remarkable achievements and successes are the result of clinical preparation and monitoring, and heart rate has played an integral role in all this. Heart rate monitor manufacturers abound in Scandinavia, and we are now witnessing a revolution in monitors and training, such as 24-hour heart rate recovery. The availability of 24-hour monitors has introduced the long overdue concept of recovery training. The ability to monitor constantly allows athletes to adjust their training to ensure appropriate rest and recovery, and, if the data suggest, to institute a change in the daily exercise plan. Record keeping is vital to this process.

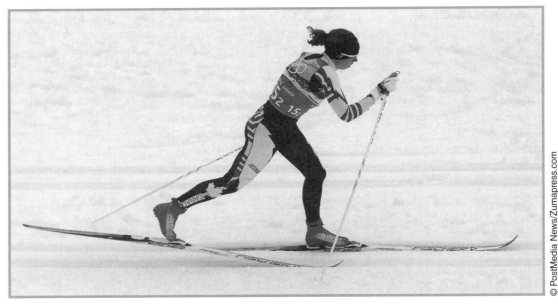

© PostMedia News/Zumapress.com

Elite cross-country skiers score very high on fitness tests. They rely heavily on intelligent heart rate training to improve their performances.

Classifying Your Current Fitness Level

To determine your baseline endurance level, use the running $\dot{V}O_2$max test from chapter 10 on running (page 127) or the maximum heart rate (MHR) assessment described in chapter 2 (page 24). For the most part, it is easier to do this while running, although it is more accurate when done skiing, especially if you want to collect MHR data at the same time. If you use the protocol outlined in chapter 10 for running, you will be able to get both a fitness classification and a maximum heart rate. Once you have this information, classify your fitness level using the maximum oxygen consumption tables in chapter 10 (table 10.2 or table 10.3, page 128) and chapter 14 (table 14.2 or table 14.3, page 180). This will also indicate which level you should start at—level 1, 2, or 3.

Determining Your Cross-Country Skiing Training Zones

The skiing test for determining MHR can be done running or on roller skis.

Sample Skiing Test for MHR

1. Find a running track or a small and gradual incline that goes for about 400 to 600 meters. If you are going to perform the test on roller skis, be sure to select an appropriate surface. Put on your heart rate monitor.

2. Do a good 0.5- to 1-mile (0.8 to 1.6 km) warm-up.

3. Perform one lap or one incline lap as fast as you can. Check the heart rate number on the monitor.

4. Take a 2-minute recovery walk or run and then repeat the run. Check the heart rate number on the monitor.

5. Take a 2-minute recovery and repeat the run again. Your heart rate at the end of this third trial will be a pretty good indicator of your MHR.

Choosing a Training Program

Cross-country skiing, like swimming and rowing, has a highly technical component. As with the other sports, we present three progressions. Level 1 is 10K, level 2 is 25K, and level 3 is a faster 25K. If you are a novice competitor, you should start at level 1 and progress to level 3. If you are more experienced, you may begin at level 2 or 3, provided that you meet the requirements of the preceding level comfortably.

The fitness test provides an objective basic fitness classification. The programs progress through the four phases of training with the specific focus on aerobic fitness in the early phases and progressing to stamina, economy, and speed, which is more anaerobic.

Level 1 is exclusively endurance focused; all work is EZ. In level 2, both distance and intensity increase and the workouts address both endurance (EZ) and stamina (MO). In level 3, you will see a noticeable difference with many more high-intensity workouts, including continuous high-level work and intervals. The focus is on economy (FA) and speed endurance (VF). Much of this work is anaerobic, focusing on speed and power workouts.

One slight difference between cross-country skiing and other exercise modes is that snow is needed for skiing. In addition, you need groomed trails so you can ski with varying degrees of intensity. Given Mother Nature's unpredictability, consider that you will need to do dry-land training often. For that reason, we provide the options for you to do all workouts running, skiing, or roller-skiing. On days when you can't snow-ski, roller-skiing is preferable to running.

As with previous programs, we use the standard heart rate data chart. You will have to calculate your own heart rate data (bpm). The ranges of percentage of MHR are shown in table 15.2.

TABLE 15.2 Cross-Country Skiing Training Phases

Training phase	Percent MHR
Phase I: Endurance (EZ)	60–75%
Phase II: Stamina (MO)	75–85%
Phase III: Economy (FA)	85–95%
Phase IV: Speed endurance (VF)	95–100%

Level 1

The goal of the level 1 training program (table 15.3) is to build up to a 10K. The focus is on endurance development, so all training sessions are at phase I, endurance (EZ). Keep in mind that at this level everything is slow and easy to allow you to comfortably develop your cardiorespiratory system and create the aerobic, or endurance, foundation you need before moving on to higher-intensity work. This is in line with the basic concept of slow progression that we outlined in chapter 8.

Level 2

The goal of the level 2 training program (table 15.4) is to build up to a 25K using variables of endurance (EZ) and stamina (MO) training. The focus is on improving the endurance built in the level 1 training program and developing stamina. It follows the principles of progression by adding slight increases in both intensity and duration with the goal of increasing your abilities over the longer distances and helping you continue to build on the endurance base. Stamina becomes important here because the step up to 25K is considerable; depending on the terrain, it may take one to two-and-a-half hours longer to do 25K versus 10K.

TABLE 15.3 Level 1 Cross-Country Skiing Training Program*

Week	Mon.	Tues.	Wed.	Thurs.	Fri.	Sat.	Sun.
1	EZ 20:00	Rest	EZ 20:00	Rest	Rest	EZ 30:00	Rest
2	EZ 20:00	Rest	EZ 20:00	Rest	Rest	EZ 30:00	Rest
3	EZ 30:00	Rest	EZ 30:00	Rest	Rest	EZ 40:00	Rest
4	EZ 30:00	Rest	EZ 30:00	Rest	Rest	EZ 40:00	Rest
5	EZ 40:00	Rest	EZ 40:00	Rest	Rest	EZ 50:00	Rest
6	EZ 40:00	Rest	EZ 40:00	Rest	Rest	EZ 50:00	Rest
7	EZ 50:00	Rest	EZ 50:00	Rest	Rest	EZ 60:00	Rest
8	EZ 50:00	Rest	EZ 30:00	Rest	Rest	Race 10K	Rest

*Goal 10k
Ski all training sessions. If weather prohibits skiing, either roller-ski or run the training session.
EZ: Heart rate zone 1.

TABLE 15.4 Level 2 Cross-Country Skiing Training Program*

Week	Mon.	Tues.	Wed.	Thurs.	Fri.	Sat.	Sun.
1	EZ 50:00	Rest	EZ 50:00	MO 20:00	Rest	EZ 60:00	Rest
2	EZ 50:00	Rest	EZ 50:00	MO 20:00	Rest	EZ 60:00	Rest
3	EZ 60:00	Rest	EZ 60:00	MO 20:00	Rest	EZ 70:00	Rest
4	EZ 60:00	Rest	EZ 60:00	MO 20:00	Rest	EZ 70:00	Rest
5	EZ 70:00	Rest	EZ 70:00	MO 30:00	Rest	EZ 80:00	Rest
6	EZ 70:00	Rest	EZ 70:00	MO 30:00	Rest	EZ 80:00	Rest
7	80:00 (EZ 50:00 and MO 30:00)	Rest	EZ 80:00	MO 30:00	Rest	EZ 90:00	Rest
8	80:00 (EZ 50:00 and MO 30:00)	Rest	EZ 80:00	MO 30:00	Rest	EZ 100:00	Rest
9	90:00 (EZ 60:00 and MO 30:00)	Rest	EZ 90:00	MO 30:00	Rest	EZ 110:00	Rest
10	100:00 (EZ 60:00 and MO 40:00)	Rest	EZ 100:00	MO 40:00	Rest	EZ 120:00	Rest
11	80:00 (EZ 50:00 and MO 30:00)	Rest	EZ 80:00	MO 30:00	Rest	EZ 120:00	Rest
12	Rest	EZ 80:00	MO 30:00	Rest	Rest	Race 25K	Rest

*Goal 25k
Ski all training sessions. If weather prohibits skiing, either roller-ski or run the training session.
EZ: Heart rate zone 1.
MO: Heart rate zone 2.

Level 3

The goal of the level 3 training program (table 15.5) is to train to complete the 25K more quickly. The focus is on improving economy and speed endurance with sessions in all four training phases (EZ, MO, FA, and VF). You'll notice an increase in intensity and the introduction of intervals and more speed sessions. Level 3 builds on the work accomplished in the level 1 and level 2 programs but adds the increased focus on intensity to help you improve your performance as opposed to just covering the distance.

Week	Mon.	Tues.	Wed.	Thurs.	Fri.	Sat.	Sun.
TABLE 15.5 Level 3 Cross-Country Skiing Training Program							
1	10K TT	Rest	EZ 50:00	FA 30:00	Rest	MO 60:00	Rest
2	A1 60:00	Rest	EZ 50:00	FA 30:00	Rest	MO 60:00	Rest
3	A1 60:00	Rest	EZ 60:00	FA 30:00	Rest	MO 60:00	Rest
4	A1 60:00	Rest	EZ 60:00	FA 30:00	Rest	MO 60:00	Rest
5	A2 88:00	Rest	EZ 70:00	A3 55:00	Rest	EZ 80:00	Rest
6	A2 88:00	Rest	EZ 70:00	A3 55:00	Rest	EZ 80:00	Rest
7	A2 88:00	Rest	EZ 80:00	A3 55:00	Rest	EZ 90:00	Rest
8	A2 88:00	Rest	EZ 80:00	A3 55:00	Rest	EZ 90:00	Rest
9	FA 30:00	Rest	EZ 90:00	A2 88:00	Rest	EZ 100:00	Rest
10	FA 30:00	Rest	EZ 10:00	A2 88:00	Rest	EZ 110:00	Rest
11	FA 30:00	Rest	EZ 80:00	A2 88:00	Rest	EZ 120:00	Rest
12	Rest	EZ 80:00	MO 30:00	Rest	Rest	Race 25K	Rest

Ski all training sessions. If weather prohibits skiing, either roller-ski or run the training session. See the chapter text for descriptions of the intervals.

KEY:
TT: Time trial
EZ: Heart rate zone 1
MO: Heart rate zone 2
FA: Heart rate zone 3

The intervals noted in table 15.5 are described here:

A1 Interval

Approximately 60:00

Warm-up: EZ 15:00

MO 10:00

EZ 5:00

FA 5:00

EZ 5:00

VF 5:00

EZ 5:00

Max effort 2:00

Cool-down: EZ 8:00

A2 Interval

Approximately 88:00

Warm-up: EZ 15:00

Max effort 2:00 followed by EZ 5:00; perform five times

Max effort 1:00 followed by EZ 5:00; perform five times

Cool-down: EZ 8:00

A3 Interval

Approximately 53:00

Warm-up: EZ 15:00

MO 30:00 with 10 × 0:20 accelerations each 2:00

Cool-down: EZ 8:00

Continuing Your Training

Progressing through these three training programs will establish a solid fitness foundation. At this point, you will want to decide whether you desire further improvements in performance or want to try longer distances. Continued improvements in performance will require you to refocus your training approach to include even higher-intensity work over both shorter and longer distances. You will also have to participate in more structured events for racing experience. If longer distances are your next objective, you will have to back off on the intensity and increase the distances noted in the level 2 program to further enhance your cardiorespiratory system and your ability to use fat as a fuel source. Before making these moves, you will need a careful evaluation of your current fitness level, so revisiting the fitness assessments would be wise. This will give you a fresh look at your current fitness, which will allow you to determine a more appropriate starting point. At this stage, you might look for some individual coaching.

CHAPTER 16

Team Sports

Coaches of team sports understand that their athletes need a foundation of conditioning to play at the highest possible levels. That's why baseball has spring training workouts and American football players suffer through conditioning sessions in the summer heat and humidity. As in endurance sports, the fitness challenges in team sports vary tremendously among sports and positions within sports. For example, the soccer player may run upward of 6 miles (9.6 km) during a 90-minute game, whereas the offensive tackle in American football may cover only a few hundred meters in a game. Regardless, all team sport athletes need an element of aerobic conditioning, because that is what governs the recovery from anaerobic activity.

Clearly, getting in shape helps team sport athletes play well. The coaches who understand this universal principle also believe in the value of breaking down the game's movements and overall abilities into sets of microskills that players can practice over and over. For our purposes, let's consider physical fitness a skill that can be broken down into parts that can be practiced separately, just like running pass routes, shooting free throws, and pitching splitters.

Before we go much further, we'd like to address briefly the issue of using heart rate monitoring while weightlifting. Weightlifting is an integral part of the conditioning routine of most athletes, and as such needs to be monitored like any other fitness routine. However, monitoring heart rate while weight training for strength or power is not reliable. Lifting weights causes large increases in blood pressure, reduces breathing frequency, and requires large static muscle contractions. The result is a blunted heart rate response to an immediate bout of exercise. For this reason, we do not advocate the use of heart rate monitoring to guide intensity while doing heavy resistance training.

Fitness Components in Team Sports

Physiologists know that physical fitness has components that can be practiced as separate skills. Applying this idea to team sports that involve constant running, such as American football, basketball, soccer, lacrosse, and rugby, we can see that athletes in these sports need the following:

- The ability to stay fast for the entire game (endurance)
- The ability to sprint back and forth for several plays in a row (stamina)
- The leg speed to be the first to get to the ball or ball carrier (speed)
- The ability to recover between exercise bouts and then repeat them over again (aerobic recovery)
- The strength to maintain position and resist opposition (power)

In other words, team athletes need to develop speed, endurance, and stamina, and they need to recover. In earlier chapters, we talked about how athletes in endurance sports train to develop these separate skills. This chapter addresses the general principles you need to understand if you play or coach a team sport.

Endurance is the foundation for all other levels of fitness. The greater your degree of endurance, the longer you can perform at a high level of effort, hopefully right up to the end of the game. To develop endurance, you need to jog slowly in the surprisingly easy effort zone of 60 to 75 percent maximum heart rate (MHR). This should be for periods much longer than most coaches require, probably for the same length as a game.

Stamina is the capacity to race up and down the court or back and forth on the field for at least a few minutes of nonstop huffing and puffing. This should not be so difficult that you have to slow down or have a sub so you can retreat to the bench for a breather. To develop stamina,

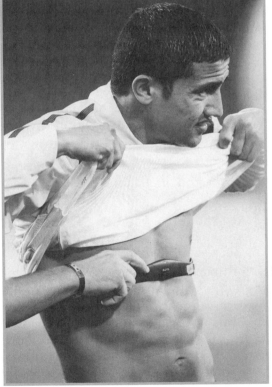

© AP Photo/Andrew Brownbill

Athletes in team sports such as soccer benefit from heart rate monitoring and training just as endurance athletes do.

you need to run several repeats for distances two or three times longer than the length of the field or court in the heart rate zone of 75 to 85 percent MHR with recovery intervals down to 70 percent before starting the next repeat.

Speed can be improved by performing classic wind sprints at 85 to 90 percent MHR. However, as opposed to the normal practice of running several of these in a row to improve mental toughness through exhaustive levels of fatigue, a full recovery interval should be used to reduce heart rate to less than 60 percent MHR so each repeat can be at full sprint speed. Sprinting all out from a running start over distances less than 50 yards (45.7 m) is ideal for this sort of fitness.

The best workouts to develop *power* are at 95 to 100 percent MHR. Going full speed up stadium steps or short hills for 10 to 15 seconds with wisely administered, complete, full recoveries to less than 60 percent MHR between efforts works well.

Determining Maximum Heart Rate

To get the necessary heart rate data, use the basic running test presented in chapter 2.

Running Test for MHR

1. Put on your heart rate monitor. Find a running track or a small and gradual incline that goes for about 400 to 600 meters.
2. Do a good 0.5- to 1-mile (0.8 to 1.6 km) warm-up.
3. Perform one lap or one incline lap as fast as you can. Check the number on your heart rate monitor at the end.
4. Take a 2-minute recovery walk or run, and then repeat the run.
5. Take a 2-minute recovery and repeat the run again. Your heart rate at the end of this third trial will be a pretty good indicator of your MHR.

Heart Rate Monitoring and Training in Team Sports

Unfortunately, many coaches and athletes confuse workouts to improve fitness skills with those to improve mental toughness. An old adage of ours is: Anyone can make an athlete tired, but not everyone can make him better. Endurance laps around the field often turn into races that athletes hope will impress the coach. What is often missing in these workouts is individualization that gives all athletes the opportunity to improve. The one-size-fits-all philosophy doesn't work because some athletes will work very hard while others are in cruise control and achieving little real adaptation.

Individualizing workouts by using heart rate data helps keep skill development sessions from turning into efforts that are much harder than necessary. For example, an off-season program for developing endurance is often implemented by a time trial that requires the athlete to run, say, 2 miles (3.2 km) in 16 minutes or faster. This simply sabotages the purpose of the workouts, because for some athletes that pace may take an effort much higher than the standard endurance zone of 60 to 75 percent MHR. Either they fail, or they have to generate efforts way above the standards required for the development of endurance.

Because endurance is the capacity to keep moving no matter how much you slow down before having to walk, you should be tested by seeing whether you can jog 3 or 4 miles (4.8 or 6.4 km) without walking. Having to meet an arbitrary standard in a time trial may force you to work harder than necessary and, in the process, risk injury or burnout. Once you have established a good base of endurance, you can maintain it with just one long jog per week. For typical off-season endurance guidelines, see the jogging section in chapter 10.

Next, you can do interval workouts at running paces designed to elevate your heart rate into a special stamina-development zone of 75 to 85 percent MHR. Two or three times a week a workout of running half a lap around the track or field several times (6 or 8 × 200 meters) with a half-lap jog to recover would be perfect for developing the stamina you need to still be running fast after several quick trips back and forth on the court or field. (This skill is obviously just what big, heavy football linemen need when they have to run the length of the field to block or tackle an opponent.) This might be optimistic, but even half this work would be beneficial.

For enhancing your natural leg speed, the objective is not punishment with continuous gassers to the point of nausea. Once you go into oxygen debt and lactic acid accumulation, two things happen, and both are bad: muscles get pulled, or you get so tired that you have no alternative but to slow down. That is not how speed and confidence are developed. When you get tired, start to feel sorry for yourself, and then slow down, you have learned the wrong lesson. The point of any and every speed development workout is to run fast, not tired and slow.

A good workout pattern for combining all these special, complementary sets of running skills follows the classic hard/easy design. Of course, you have to work them into your game schedule, and we realize that many sports have multiple games per week. Ideally, you can use easy jogging workouts at endurance maintenance levels of 60 to 65 percent MHR to fully rest up for a game. The day after the game, easy jogging in the 65 to 70 percent MHR zone will aid recovery. The next day, stamina workouts at 75 to 85 percent MHR will fit in nicely, followed the next day by recovery jogging at 65 to 70 percent. A speed workout can then follow, then an easy recovery day, and finally, a power workout. You don't have to accomplish all this within a week or even two. Just keep following the pattern until you have accomplished the full rotation, and then begin again.

If you need mental toughness conditioning, instead of a speed or power workout, run 3 × 300 meters, running most of the last 100 meters at 100 percent MHR. The goal of this workout is to produce a full load of lactic acid from a really deep oxygen debt over the first 200 meters and then struggle down the last 100 meters. Yes, you will feel sorry and regret being there, but when mental toughness is the pure objective of a running workout, this will get the job done. But let's not confuse the issues—pure speed is not developed by slowing down. Leg speed can be enhanced by running full speed and then stopping before any fatigue sets in.

One more thought: Running should not be punishment. Running is the golden skill that allows all athletes to play at their best. Why use it to develop an aversion to the very skill that success depends on? Run for fun, or dash for cash, but do it right so that you use running to help you achieve your best. It's also for the good of your team.

Although heart rate technology traditionally has been restricted to individual endurance athletes, technologies developed in the past 10 years have extended heart rate monitoring to the team sport environment. Team telemetry systems allow coaches to observe the work efforts of 10 to 12 athletes at the same time. Using this technology, coaches can see in a heartbeat who is working harder and who is in better shape. Most important, they can use heart rate data to help athletes work out sensibly, progressively, and safely.

Whether a coach is monitoring basic fitness and conditioning or doing fitness testing, a team telemetry system is a wonderful analysis tool. It allows the coach to ensure that the fittest athletes are working hard and getting fitter, and not just doing enough to come in a few meters ahead of the least fit guys. These systems enhance accountability and individuality and are a welcome addition to the arena of heart rate monitoring. You could say that they make the playing field more even. Team telemetry heart rate systems are great for preseason and early season monitoring, as well as for gather data during game situations, giving coaches and athletes alike unique insights into the effort and heart rate responses in both training and competitive environments. And their greatest value may be in their ability to guide recovery.

APPENDIX

MHR	Percentage of maximum heart rate (MHR)								
	100%	95%	90%	85%	80%	75%	70%	65%	60%
205	205	194	184	174	164	153	143	133	123
204	204	193	183	173	163	153	142	132	122
203	203	192	182	172	162	152	142	131	121
202	202	191	181	171	161	151	141	131	121
201	201	190	180	170	160	150	140	130	120
200	200	190	180	170	160	150	140	130	120
199	199	189	179	169	159	149	139	129	119
198	198	188	178	168	158	148	138	128	118
197	197	187	177	167	157	147	137	128	118
196	196	186	176	166	156	147	137	127	117
195	195	185	175	165	156	146	136	126	117
194	194	184	174	164	155	145	135	126	116
193	193	183	173	164	154	144	135	125	115
192	192	182	172	163	153	144	134	124	115
191	191	181	171	162	152	143	133	124	114
190	190	180	171	161	152	142	133	123	114
189	189	179	170	160	151	141	132	122	113
188	188	178	169	159	150	141	131	122	112
187	187	177	168	158	149	140	130	121	112
186	186	176	167	158	148	139	130	120	111
185	185	175	166	157	148	138	129	120	111
184	184	174	165	156	147	138	128	119	110
183	183	173	164	155	146	137	128	118	109
182	182	172	163	154	145	136	127	118	109
181	181	171	162	153	144	135	126	117	108
180	180	171	162	153	144	135	126	117	108
179	179	170	161	152	143	134	125	116	107
178	178	169	160	151	142	133	124	115	106
177	177	168	159	150	141	132	123	115	106

(continued)

HEART RATE TRAINING ZONE CALCULATION CHART *(continued)*

MHR	Percentage of maximum heart rate (MHR)								
	100%	95%	90%	85%	80%	75%	70%	65%	60%
176	176	167	158	149	140	132	123	114	105
175	175	166	157	148	140	131	122	113	105
174	174	165	156	147	139	130	121	113	104
173	173	164	155	147	138	129	121	112	103
172	172	163	154	146	137	129	120	111	103
171	171	162	153	145	136	128	119	111	102
170	170	161	153	144	136	127	119	110	102
169	169	160	152	143	135	126	118	109	101
168	168	159	151	143	134	126	117	109	100
167	167	158	150	141	133	125	116	108	100
166	166	157	149	141	132	124	116	107	99
165	165	156	148	140	132	123	115	107	99
164	164	155	147	139	131	123	114	106	98
163	163	154	146	138	130	122	114	105	97
162	162	153	145	137	129	121	113	105	97
161	161	152	144	136	128	120	112	104	96
160	160	152	144	136	128	120	112	104	96
159	159	151	143	135	127	119	111	103	95
158	158	150	142	134	126	118	110	102	94
157	157	149	141	133	125	117	109	102	94
156	156	148	140	132	124	117	109	101	93
155	155	147	139	131	124	116	108	100	93
154	154	146	138	130	123	115	107	100	92
153	153	145	137	130	122	114	107	99	91
152	152	144	136	129	121	114	106	98	91
151	151	143	135	128	120	113	105	98	90
150	150	142	135	127	120	112	105	97	90
149	149	141	134	126	119	111	104	96	89
148	148	140	133	125	118	111	103	96	88
147	147	139	132	124	117	110	102	95	88
146	146	138	131	124	116	109	102	94	87
145	145	137	130	123	116	108	101	94	87

INDEX

Note: Page references followed by an italicized *f* or *t* indicate information contained in figures and tables, respectively.

A

acceleration 86, 88
Achilles' tendonitis 57
acute heart rate response 109-110
adenosine triphosphate (ATP) 47, 56
aerobic effort zone 5, 5*f*, 6*t*, 54
aerobic endurance training
    about 53-54
    and anaerobic threshold 130-131
    cross-country skiing 194, 195*t*
    cycling 148*t*
    development 56-57
    fartlek training 58-60
    increasing intensity 63
    LSD training 58, 60
    maintenance program 64-66
    physiological adaptations to 54-56
    recovery zones 66
    rowing 182-183, 182*t*
    running 132-134
    sample base-building pattern 61-63
    sample endurance enhancing pattern 64
    swimming 158*t*
    for team sports 198, 199, 200-201
    training techniques 58-60
    weight loss and 65-66
    workout duration 61
aerobic energy system 46, 48-49, 49*t*
aerobic metabolism 25-26, 50
age, and heart rate 31
American College of Sports Medicine 125, 127
anabolic training 87
anaerobic capability 52
anaerobic effort zone 5, 5*f*, 6*t*
anaerobic glycolysis energy system 46, 47-48, 49*t*
anaerobic metabolism 25-26

anaerobic threshold (AT). *See also* stamina (AT) training
    about 15
    determining heart rate at 71
    determining running 130-131
    determining swimming 157
    heart rate changes at 35-36
    and interval training 98
    lactate monitoring 95-96
    stamina development and 69-70
Armstrong, Lance 192*t*
ASCM's Guidelines for Testing and Prescription (ASCM) 127
ATP-PC energy system 47, 49*t*, 50
atrial fibrillation 32
AT training. *See* stamina (AT) training

B

blood lactate profiling 95
blood volume changes 55
Borg Scale of Perceived Exertion 8-9, 26

C

calorie expenditure 41
carbohydrate 50, 51, 56, 99
cardiac creep 32-34, 33*f*
cardiac crimp 34
cardiovascular drift 32-34, 33*f*, 98
catabolic training 87
century ride training program 152-153, 152*t*, 153*t*
chronic heart rate 110-111
Connolly-Benson stress test for walkers 118
creatine phosphate 47
cross-country skiing
    about training 191-192, 192*t*
    aerobic *vs.* anaerobic energy usage 46*t*
    current fitness level 193

cross-country skiing *(continued)*
   heart rate training zones 193
   tempo workouts 73
   training phases 194*t*
   training programs 193-197, 194*t,*
      195*t*, 196*t*
cycling
   about training 143-145
   aerobic *vs.* anaerobic energy use 46*t*
   century ride training program 152-
      153, 152*t*, 153*t*
   current fitness level 145, 146*t*, 147*t*
   heart rate training zones 147
   tempo workouts 73
   training phases 145*t*
   training programs 147-153, 148*t*,
      149*t*, 150*t*, 151*t*, 152*t*, 153*t*

D
Daehlie, Bjorn 192*t*
dehydration 32-33
duration of workouts 105

E
economy 4, 5*f*, 6*t*
economy training
   activities for enhancing 78-82
   cross-country skiing 196-197, 196*t*
   cycling 149*t*, 150*t*
   fartlek training 78-79
   interval training 79-82, 83
   physiological adaptations to economy
      training 76
   rowing 186-189, 187*t*
   sample pattern for enhancing 82-83
   swimming 161-164, 162*t*
   transition to enhancing economy 77-
      78
efficiency 77
effort, understanding 8-9
effort zones 5, 5*f*, 6*t*, 54
emotional changes 35
endocrine system adaptations 68
endurance, aerobic 4, 5*f*, 6*t*
endurance training, aerobic
   about 53-54
   and anaerobic threshold 130-131
   cross-country skiing 194, 195*t*
   cycling 148*t*
   development 56-57
   fartlek training 58-60
   increasing intensity 63
   LSD training 58, 60

maintenance program 64-66
   physiological adaptations to 54-56
   recovery zones 66
   rowing 182-183, 182*t*
   running 132-134
   sample base-building pattern 61-63
   sample endurance enhancing pattern
      64
   swimming 158*t*
   for team sports 198, 199, 200-201
   training techniques 58-60
   weight loss and 65-66
   workout duration 61
energy expenditure 16, 19-20
energy production systems 46-52, 46*t*,
   49*t*
ergometers, indoor rowing 178
exertion, perceived. *See* rate of perceived
   exertion (RPE)

F
fartlek training 58-60, 72, 78-79
fast-twitch muscle fibers 7, 50, 51-52, 96
fat 51, 57
Faulkner test 54
fitness, physical
   components of 4-6, 5*f*
   components of team sports 199-200
   cross-country skiing assessment 193
   cycling assessment 145, 146*t*, 147*t*
   goals and personalization of 6-7, 8
   and maximum heart rate changes 55
   rowing assessment 179-180, 179*t*,
      180*t*
   running and jogging assessment 127-
      129, 128*t*
   swimming assessment 155-156
   walking assessment 116-117, 117*t*
fitness testing 23-24, 28
fitness testing errors 23-24
5K training program 136-137, 138*t*
flexibility 76
football 50
form, mechanics and 88, 97
frequency of workouts 105
fuel sources, HR zone 6*t*

G
gender, and heart rate 7, 30, 31-32
genetic makeup 7
glycogen 66
glycogen deficit 57
glycolytic energy system 46, 47-48, 49*t*

H

half Ironman-distance triathlon 166-167, 167*t*, 168, 168*t*, 174, 175*t*, 176*t*
half-marathon training program 140, 141*t*
heart rate. *See also* maximum heart rate
  about 3-4, 9-11, 10*f*
  acute heart rate response 109-110
  at anaerobic threshold (AT) 35-36, 71
  cardiac stress testing 24
  changes in maximum 55
  chronic heart rate 110-111
  determining maximum 24-25, 26-27
  factors affecting 30-35, 33*f*
  fitness testing errors 23-24
  frequent self-testing of 35-36
  improved stroke volume 18, 23, 30-31, 55, 111
  information from 9
  Karvonen formula 26-27
  and multisport athletes 24, 28
  predicting maximum 22-23
  resting heart rate 7, 10-11, 10*f*, 30-31
  running maximum 129-130
  swimming maximum 156-157
  variability across exercise modes 24
  within-exercise recovery 109-110
heart rate reserve (HRR) 27
heart rate training zones
  calculating 25-29, 203-204
  cross-country skiing 193
  cycling 147
  effort zones 5, 5*f*, 6*t*, 54
  fuel sources for 6*t*
  recovery zones 66
  rowing 181
  running and jogging 131
  swimming 157-158
  triathlon 167, 167*t*, 169, 169*t*
  walking 119
heart size 7
hemodilution 55
high-intensity, continuous exercise (HICE) 92, 94-96
hitting the wall 57
hockey 46*t*
hormonal changes 35

I

iliotibial band syndrome 57
Indurain, Miguel 30, 192*t*
injuries, overuse 57, 60, 68, 89, 126
intensity of workouts 19, 105

interval training 73, 79-82, 83, 96-98, 97*t*, 109-110, 201. *See also* fartlek training
Ironman-distance triathlon 166-167, 167*t*, 168, 168*t*

J

jogging. *See* running and jogging

K

Karvonen formula 26-27
Kristiannssen, Ingrid 192*t*

L

lactate threshold (LT). *See also* stamina (AT) training
  about 15
  determining heart rate at 71
  determining running 130-131
  determining swimming 157
  heart rate changes at 35-36
  and interval training 98
  lactate monitoring 95-96
  stamina development and 69-70
lactic acid buildup 59, 69-70, 95-96
lactic acid system 46, 47-48, 49*t*
lead legs 34-35
LeMond, Greg 192*t*
long, slow distance (LSD) training 58, 60

M

maintenance, exercise 106
marathons 46*t*, 57
marathon training program 140-141, 142*t*
maximum heart rate. *See also* heart rate
  about 10
  changes with fitness level 55
  determining 24-25, 26-27
  determining running 129-130
  determining swimming 156-157
  fitness testing errors 23-24
  Karvonen formula 26-29
  in power and speed training 86
  predicting 22-23
  and team sports 200
  variability across exercise modes 24, 28
mechanics and form 88, 97
mental toughness 77, 88-89, 201-202
mesocycles 107
microcycles 107
1-mile walking test 117, 117*t*
mitochondria 56

mode of workouts 105
monitors, heart rate
    choosing 42
    fitting and proper use of 37-39
    innovations in 41-42
    technical difficulties of 39-41
Moses, Edwin 91
Mota, Rosa 192*t*
multisport athletes, and heart rate 24, 28
muscle fiber types 7, 50, 51-52, 96
muscle recovery 10
muscles
    changes with aerobic training 55
    changes with speed and power
        training 88
    changes with stamina training 76
    muscle fiber types 7, 50, 51-52, 96
    muscle recovery 10
musculoskeletal adaptations 57, 68, 76

N
NSAIDS 126
nutrition
    and energy supply systems 46, 50, 52
    overtraining and overreaching 111,
        112
    in speed and power training 87, 89
    in stamina training 69, 73

O
Olympic-distance triathlon 166-167,
        167*t*, 168, 168*t*, 171, 172*t*, 173*t*
1-mile walking test 117, 117*t*
overload, exercise 105-106, 115
overtraining and overreaching
    avoiding 111-112
    lead legs 34-35
oxidative system. *See* aerobic energy
        system
oxygen consumption (VO2)
    changes with aerobic training 55
    cross-country ski data 13*t*, 191, 192*t*
    in cycling 143
    cycling data 14*t*, 17*t*
    estimated by heart rate 5
    heart rate *vs.* 16*f*
    MHR–VO2max conversion 12*t*
    and muscle fiber composition 7
    slow-twitch muscle fibers and 51
    VO2 and heart rate 11-18, 12*t*, 13*t*,
        14*t*, 16*f*, 17*f*, 17*t*
    VO2max 11, 54, 143, 191, 192*t*

P
pace running 92, 94-96
perceived exertion. *See* rate of perceived
        exertion (RPE)
periodization of training 107-108
physical fitness. *See* fitness, physical
plantar fasciitis 57
positive splits 82-83
power training. *See* speed and power
        training
Prefontaine, Steve 192*t*
progressive resistance 108-109

R
rate of perceived exertion (RPE)
    Benson chart 29, 30*t*
    Borg scale 8-9, 26
recovery
    glycogen deficit 57
    monitoring training progress and 109-
        112
    and resting heart rate 11, 31
    in speed and power training 99-100,
        100*t*
recovery zones 66
respiratory adaptations 55
resting heart rate 7, 10-11, 10*f*, 30-31,
        110-111
reversibility, exercise 106
rowing
    about training 178
    aerobic *vs.* anaerobic energy usage
        46*t*, 50
    current fitness level 179-180, 179*t*,
        180*t*
    heart rate training zones 181
    HICE session 96
    tempo workouts 73
    training programs 181-189, 182*t*,
        184*t*, 187*t*
running and jogging
    about 125-127
    building endurance 132-134
    competitive running 136-142, 138*t*,
        139*t*, 141*t*, 142*t*
    current fitness level 127-129, 128*t*
    determining anaerobic threshold 130-
        131
    determining maximum heart rate 129-
        130
    energy sources for 49*t*
    5K training program 136-137, 138*t*

half-marathon training program 140, 141*t*

heart rate training zones 131

marathon training program 140-141, 142*t*

recreational running 134, 135*t*

running test for MHR 25, 29, 30*t*

for team sports 199-202

10K training program 137-140, 139*t*

training programs 131-142 , 135*t*, 138*t*, 139*t*, 141*t*, 142*t*

year-long periodization 114*t*

S

skiing, cross-country. *See* cross-country skiing

slow-twitch muscle fibers 7, 50, 51-52

soccer 46*t*, 50, 198

specificity, exercise 106

speed, about 4-5, 5*f*, 6, 6*t*

speed and power training

about 85-87

cross-country skiing 196-197, 196*t*

cycling 149*t*, 150*t*

high-intensity, continuous exercise (HICE) 92, 94-96

interval training 96-98, 97*t*

physiological adaptations to 88-89

recovery during 99-100, 100*t*

rowing 186-189, 187*t*

sample workouts 90-91, 90*t*

speed and power development 89-92, 90*t*

swimming 161-164, 162*t*

for team sports 200, 201

training techniques 92-98

transition to 92

workout pattern for 99

sprinting 46*t*, 52

sprint triathlon 166-167, 167*t*, 168, 168*t*, 169, 170*t*, 171*t*

stamina 4, 5*f*, 6*t*

stamina (AT) training

about 67-68

benefit of 70, 131

cross-country skiing 194-195, 195*t*

cycling 149*t*, 150*t*

developing stamina 72-74

economy development 76-77

fartlek training 72

AT heart rate 71

interval training 73

physiological adaptations to 68-69

physiological adaptations to economy training 76

rowing 184-186, 184*t*

sample improvement pattern 74-76

stamina development 69-70

swimming 159-161, 159*t*

for team sports 199-200, 201

tempo workouts 72-73

transition to 71-72

transition to enhancing economy 77-78

stress fractures 57

stroke volume, improved 18, 23, 30-31, 111

swimming

about training 154-155

aerobic *vs.* anaerobic energy usage 46*t*

current fitness level 155-156

determining anaerobic threshold 157

heart rate training zones 157-158

maximum heart rate 156-157

tempo workouts 73

training programs 157-165, 158*t*, 159*t*, 162*t*, 164*t*

T

target heart rate training zones. *See* heart rate training zones

team sports

fitness components of 199-200

heart rate training and 8-9, 198, 200-202

maximum heart rate 200

temperature, and heart rate 31, 32-34

tempo workouts 72-73, 94

10K training program 137-140, 139*t*

Tour de France 143

track events energy sources 49*t*

training programs. *See also specific sports and activities*

about 103-104

and energy production systems 46-52, 46*t*, 49*t*

factors in designing 104-107

individualizing objectives 8

monitoring progress and recovery 109-112

periodization 107-108

principles of progressive resistance 108-109

putting factors together 113-114, 113*f*, 114*t*

sport-specificity 45-46

training zones, heart rate
  calculating 25-29
  cross-country skiing 193
  cycling 147
  effort zones 5, 5*f*, 6*t*, 54
  fuel sources for 6*t*
  recovery zones 66
  rowing 181
  running and jogging 131
  swimming 157-158
  triathlon 167, 167*t*, 169, 169*t*
  walking 119
triathlon
  about training 166-167
  half-Ironman training 174, 175*t*, 176*t*
  heart rate training zones 167, 167*t*,
    169, 169*t*
  Olympic-distance training 171, 172*t*,
    173*t*
  race distances 166-167, 167*t*
  sprint-distance training 169, 170*t*,
    171*t*
  swimming 164-165, 164*t*
  training programs 168-169, 168*t*, 169*t*
24-hour monitoring 41

V
ventilatory threshold. *See* anaerobic
    threshold (AT)

VO2 (oxygen consumption)
  changes with aerobic training 55
  cross-country ski data 13*t*, 191, 192*t*
  in cycling 143
  cycling data 14*t*, 17*t*
  estimated by heart rate 5
  and heart rate 11-18, 12*t*, 13*t*, 14*t*, 16*f*,
    17*f*, 17*t*
  heart rate *vs.* 16*f*
  MHR–VO2max conversion 12*t*
  and muscle fiber composition 7
  relationship to heart rate 11-18, 12*t*,
    13*t*, 14*t*, 16*f*, 17*f*, 17*t*
  slow-twitch muscle fibers and 51
  VO2max 11, 54, 143, 191, 192*t*

W
walking
  about 115-116
  current fitness level 116-117, 117*t*
  determining maximum heart rate 117-
    118
  heart rate training zones 119
  training program for 119-124
weightlifting 198

ABOUT THE AUTHORS

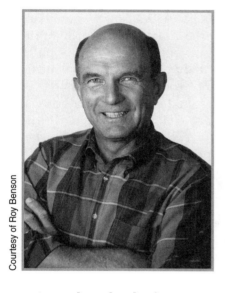

Courtesy of Roy Benson

Roy T. Benson, MPE, CFI, is an exercise scientist and distance-running coach. He has run competitively for more than 40 years, and he has coached professionally for 46 years for military, club, university, and high school teams. From 1993 to 2008, his boys' and girls' cross-country teams at Marist High School in Atlanta, Georgia, won a total of 16 state championships, and his cross-country and track runners won 21 individual state titles. Benson is also the owner and president of Running, Ltd., a company that has been operating Nike-sponsored summer camps for both adult and high school runners since 1973.

Benson has been a consultant about heart rate training for both Polar and Nike and has written three books for runners on the subject. He also serves as a special contributor to *Running Times* magazine and has been a contributing editor for *Running Journal* magazine. His booklet *Precision Running*, published by Polar Electro, has sold over 200,000 copies and has been translated into seven languages. Sales of *Coach Benson's Secret Workouts* book have reached more than 7,000. Benson lives on Amelia Island, Florida.

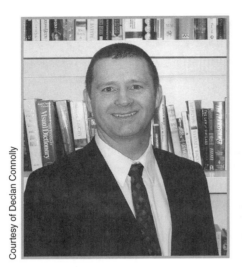

Courtesy of Declan Connolly

Dr. Declan Connolly, FACSM, CSCS, is a professor and exercise physiologist at the University of Vermont where he is also director of the Human Performance Laboratory. He consults to numerous sports organizations including the National Hockey League, the National Football League, U.S. Rowing, and U.S. Skiing and has served as a consultant to the International Olympic Committee on several occasions. In addition to more than 300 publications in scientific journals, his work is widely quoted in the popular media, including stories in the *New York Times*, *Los Angeles Times*, *London Times*, *Runner's World*, *Prevention*, *Health*, and *Self.* His work appears on more than 24,000 Web sites and has been the subject of news stories on Fox, BBC, CBS, and numerous other TV and radio networks.

Connolly is a lifelong exerciser and athlete, boasting several national cycling championships as a school boy in his native Ireland. More recently he has turned his focus to triathlon and Ironman competitions. Connolly lives in Burlington, Vermont. His Web site is www.vermontfit.com.

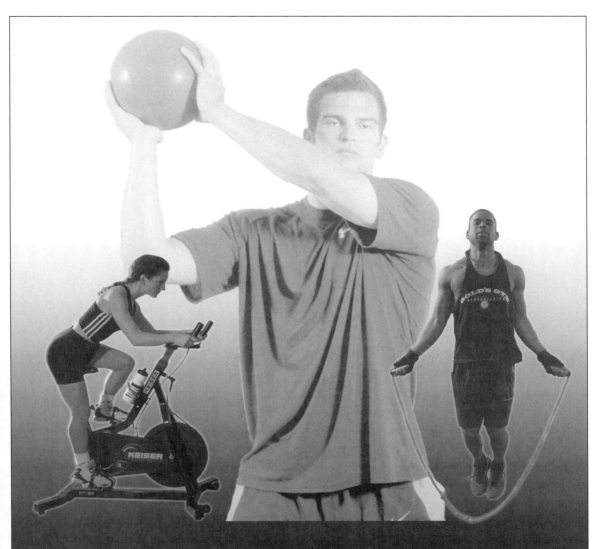

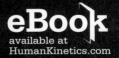